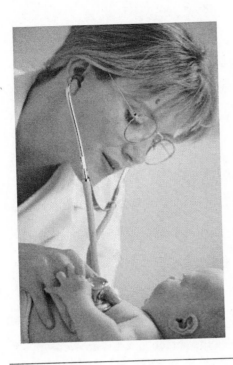

BARKLEY'S REVIEW GUIDE

for

Pediatric Nurse Practitioners

Thomas W. Barkley, Jr., DSN, ACNP-BC

President
Barkley & Associates, Inc.
West Hollywood, California

and

Professor
Director of Graduate and Nurse Practitioner Programs
California State University, Los Angeles
School of Nursing
Los Angeles, California

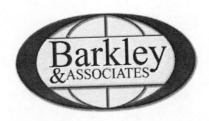

Barkley & Associates, Inc.

P.O. Box 69901
West Hollywood, CA 90069

Notice

Pediatric nursing and the practice of pediatric nurse practitioners is an ever-changing field. Standard safety precautions must be followed, but as new research and clinical experience broaden our knowledge, changes in treatment and drug therapy may become necessary or appropriate. Readers are advised to check the most current product information provided by the manufacturer of each drug to be administered to verify the recommended dose, the method and duration of administration and contraindications. It is the responsibility of the licensed prescriber, relying on expertise and knowledge of the patient, to determine dosages and the best treatment for each individual patient. Neither Barkley & Associates nor any contributing authors assume any responsibility for any injury and/or damage to persons or property arising from this publication.

Thomas W. Barkley, Jr., DSN, ACNP-BC
President
Barkley & Associates, Inc.

International Standard Book Number 978-0-615-45979-0

Printed in the United States of America

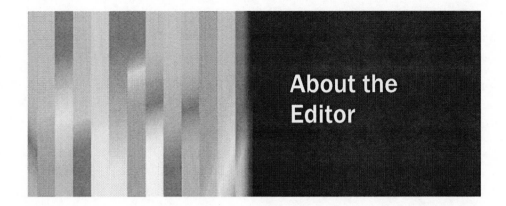

About the Editor

Thomas W. Barkley, Jr., DSN, ACNP-BC is President of Barkley & Associates, Inc., dedicated to providing the nation's best nurse practitioner certification review/clinical update and continuing education courses. He is also a Professor of Nursing and Director of Graduate and Nurse Practitioner Programs at California State University, Los Angeles. Since the mid-1990s, Dr. Barkley has been actively teaching, developing, and implementing nurse practitioner continuing education offerings both nationally and internationally.

Dr. Barkley's clinical background and practice are in critical and acute care nursing, where he holds national certification as an acute care nurse practitioner from the American Nurses Credentialing Center. He received a bachelor of science in nursing degree from the University of Alabama, a master's degree in critical care nursing from the University of Virginia, and holds the doctor of science in nursing degree with a specialty in nursing education and nursing education administration from the University of Alabama at Birmingham.

In addition to his classroom and practice responsibilities, Dr. Barkley is the primary editor of the American Journal of Nursing Book-of-the-Year award-winning text, *Practice Guidelines for Acute Care Nurse Practitioners*. He has also published numerous refereed articles related to acute care nursing practice, nursing education, and multicultural HIV/AIDS prevention.

Using expertise gleaned from his years of experience, Dr. Barkley has assisted thousands of nurse practitioners with successful passing of their initial national certification exams. Additionally, his company offers the most extensive number of different certification review/clinical update courses in the country serving nurse practitioners in the following specialties: pediatrics, family, adult, acute care, gerontological, adult/gerontological, psychiatric/mental health, and women's health.

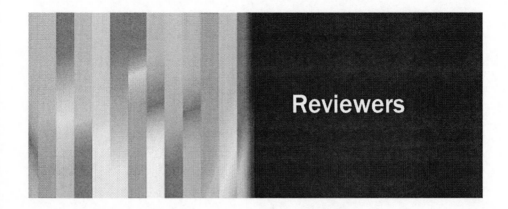

Reviewers

Kathleen P. Wilson, DSN, PNP-BC, FNP-BC, CPNP
Nurse Practitioner – Private Practice
Pediatrics and Internal Medicine
Tallahassee, Florida
Contributing Faculty – Graduate Program
Walden University
School of Nursing

Joetta D. Wallace, MSN, CPON, FNP-C
Nurse Practitioner – Pediatrics
Coordinator, Pediatric Palliative Care Program
Miller Children's Hospital
Long Beach, California
Associate Clinical Professor, Department of Pediatrics
University of Southern California
Los Angeles, California

Sara Majors, PhD, DNP, CPNP
Associate Clinical Professor
Advanced Pediatric Health
University of South Alabama
College of Nursing
Mobile, Alabama

Cynthia B. Hughes, EdD, PNP-BC
Professor
Director of the School of Nursing
California State University, Los Angeles
Los Angeles, California

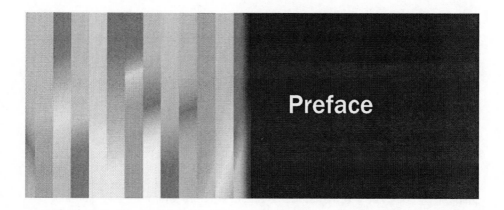

Preface

Barkley's Review Guide for Pediatric Nurse Practitioners is designed as a streamlined reference text for both pediatric and family nurse practitioners working with children of all ages. The objective of this work was to fill a void in the marketplace by offering a book without superfluous pictures, graphs and charts, while providing timely and essential information needed for prudent decision-making in pediatric clinical practice.

Utilizing national pediatric experts along with national certification examination content blueprint outlines from the American Nurses Credentialing Center (ANCC) and the Pediatric Nursing Certification Board (PNCB), the text offers a comprehensive look at the most common pediatric diagnoses and practice considerations. Whether preparing for an initial national certification exam or needing an all inclusive, evidence-based update of the latest pediatric practice guidelines and trends, the book is ideal.

Designed in a detailed, yet easy to read, quick to find, outline format, *Barkley's Review Guide for Pediatric Nurse Practitioners* is divided into three sections. Section I: Pediatric Health Considerations explores common fundamental principles organized by developmental age group, including immunization recommendations. Unique to other books, this section ends with chapters addressing genetic evaluations and pediatric disaster planning.

Section II: Pediatric Issues and Disorders uses both an age appropriate and systems-specific approach to address pediatric conditions and disorders frequently encountered in clinical practice. Over 370 pages of the most common pediatric patient presentations are included, highlighted by causes/incidence data, signs/symptoms, laboratory/diagnostic considerations, and the most up-to-date management and treatment strategies.

Preface

Finally, extensively detailed unlike any other pediatric review text, the book ends with Section III: Practice Issues, Trends, and Health Policy. In this section, national implications affecting nurse practitioner practice are examined. Valuable topics for the practitioner include: scope of practice, reimbursement, regulatory and accrediting guidelines, navigating the health care system on behalf of the patient, health care policy, financing, billing and coding, regulatory and accrediting guidelines, federal and state regulations, examining and utilizing evidence in practice, and ethical principles.

With practice questions included at the end of every chapter, this book was inspired by our valued former students and customers to provide an additional pivotal resource so they may continue their successful careers. We trust that you will find the text comprehensively useful in your practice, as well.

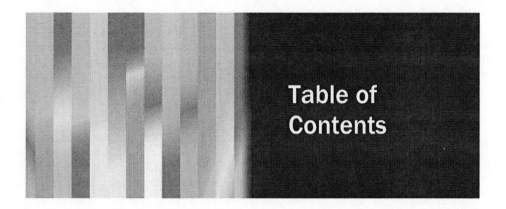

Table of Contents

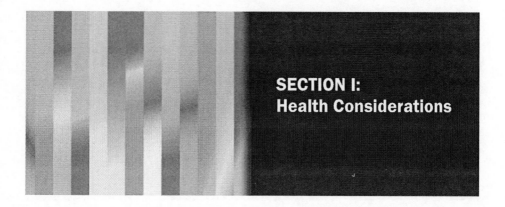

SECTION I:
Health Considerations

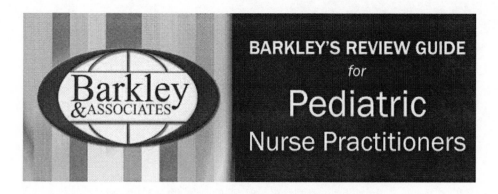

BARKLEY'S REVIEW GUIDE

for

Pediatric

Nurse Practitioners

Prenatal/Newborn Health Screening

In the evaluation of any pediatric patient, an accurate history is essential to identify potential and actual health problems. In addition to the traditional history elements including chief complaint, history of present illness, and review of systems, etc., a comprehensive history of the newborn (and to age 3 years) should include a detailed assessment of the pre/peri/postnatal course.

The Newborn Assessment: History

Prenatal History

1.   Pregnancy etiology
      a.   Intentional
      b.   Natural reproduction
      c.   In-vitro fertilization
      d.   Other infertility protocols
2.   Course of prenatal care
3.   Xenobiotics used during the gestational period
4.   Health problems during pregnancy
5.   Intrauterine fetal health problems in utero
6.   How does the mother feel about this pregnancy?

Perinatal History

1.   Vaginal delivery vs. C-section
2.   Planned vs. emergent C-section
3.   Induced labor
4.   Length of labor and delivery
5.   Gestational age at birth
6.   Style of delivery
7.   Analgesia/anesthesia
8.   Complications
      a.   Placenta previa/abruptio
      b.   Meconium
      c.   Forceps/vacuum
9.   Birth size/weight
      a.   Low birth weight (LBW): < 2500 g

  b.   Very low birth weight (VLBW): < 1,500 g
  c.   Extremely low birth weight (ELBW): < 1,000 g
10.   Assessment of weight for gestational age
  a.   Appropriate for gestational age (AGA): Between the 10th and 90th percentile
  b.   Large for gestational age (LGA): Weight > 90th percentile, associated with maternal diabetes
  c.   Small for gestational age (SGA): Weight < 10th percentile; symmetric vs. asymmetric
11.   APGAR scores (5 areas of assessment for a total of 10 points): Appearance, heart rate, grimace, activity, and breathing

APGAR Scoring

(Maximum Score at 1 and 5 minutes = 10)

APGAR Sign	2	1	0
Appearance (skin coloration)	Normal color all over (hands and feet are pink)	Normal color (but hands and feet are bluish)	Bluish-gray or pale all over
Heart Rate (pulse)	Normal (above 100 beats per minute)	Below 100 beats per minute	Absent (no pulse)
Grimace (responsiveness or "reflex irritability")	Pulls away, sneezes, or coughs with stimulation	Facial movement only (grimace) with stimulation	Absent (no response to stimulation)
Activity (muscle tone)	Active, spontaneous movement	Arms and legs flexed with little movement	No movement, "floppy" tone
Breathing (rate and effort)	Normal rate and effort, good cry	Slow or irregular breathing, weak cry	Absent (no breathing)

Postnatal History

1.   Hospital course
2.   Maternal problems
  a.   Bleeding
  b.   Volume problems
  c.   Response to anesthesia
  d.   Breastfeeding
  e.   Depression
  f.   Fever/infection

3.   Infant problems
      a.   ABO/Rh incompatibilities
      b.   Hyperbilirubinemia
      c.   Hip dysplasia
      d.   Murmurs
      e.   Talipes equinovarus congenita (club feet)
      f.   Genetic syndromes

The Newborn Assessment: Physical Examination

General

1.   Weight, length, head circumference
      a.   Average length: 20 to 21 inches (51 cm)
      b.   Average weight: 7 lbs (3.1 kg)
      c.   Average head circumference: 13 to 14 inches (33 to 35 cm)
      d.   Ethnic differences in weight:
           i.   African American infants generally weigh 181 to 240 g less than Caucasian infants
           ii.   Asian, Filipino, Hawaiian, and Puerto Rican babies also weigh less than Caucasian infants
           iii.   Native American Indian babies vary a great deal; as much as 362 g separate the mean birth weights of various tribes
2.   Assessment of gestational age: Length of gestation also has an ethnic variation
      a.   African American infants have an average of 9 days shorter gestational period as compared with Caucasian infants
      b.   African American babies are more mature than Caucasian infants at similar gestational durations
      c.   Premature African American infants have a better survival rate than premature Caucasian infants
      d.   Infants born at gestational periods 37th to 41st weeks have the best health outcomes
      e.   Those born prior to 37 weeks of gestation are premature and those born after 41 weeks of gestation are post-term
3.   Intrauterine growth retardation (IUGR)
      a.   SGA: Symmetric IUGR (33% of SGA infants)
           i.   Head circumference, weight, and length are all < 10th percentile
           ii.   Usually suggests long-term compromise to the fetus or the presence of an intrinsic problem
               1.   Genetic: Congenital or chromosomal abnormalities

5

        2.   Intrauterine infection: Viral, bacterial, protozoal, spirochete

        3.   Inborn errors of metabolism

        4.   Environmental: Drugs, nicotine, x-ray exposure

b.   SGA: Asymmetric IUGR (55% of SGA infants)

      i.   Head circumference and length within normal limits (WNL); weight < 10th percentile

      ii.   Due to acute extra fetal compromise (usually occurs > 24 weeks)

        1.   Chronic hypertension

        2.   Preeclampsia

        3.   Renal disease

        4.   Cyanotic heart disease

        5.   Hemoglobinopathies

        6.   Abruptio placentae

        7.   Multiple gestation

        8.   Altitude

4.   LGA: Weight (> 90th percentile)

a.   Maternal diabetes

b.   Beckwith-Wiedemann syndrome: Congenital (present from birth) growth disorder; causes large body size, large organs and other symptoms

c.   Hydrous fetalis: Fetal condition defined as an abnormal accumulation of fluid in two or more fetal compartments

d.   Large mother

5.   Dubowitz/Ballard Exam for Gestational Age if newborn is suspected to be SGA/LGA

a.   Physical maturity assessed within 2 hours of birth: Points from –2 to +5 given for six criteria

      i.   Skin texture: Sticky, smooth, peeling

      ii.   Lanugo: Soft downy hair on baby's body is absent in immature infants, present with maturity, and disappears with postmaturity

      iii.   Plantar creases: On sole of feet ranges from absent to covering the entire feet

      iv.   Breast: Thickness and size of breast tissue

      v.   Eyes/ears: Eyes fused or open, amount of ear cartilage present, and the amount of elastic recoil of cartilage

      vi.   Genitals

        1.   Male: Presence of testes and appearance of scrotum from smooth to wrinkled

        2.   Female: Appearance and size of clitoris and labia

      b.   Neuromuscular maturity assessed within 24 hours of birth: Points assigned to 6 measures
                  i.   Posture: How does the baby hold his/her arms and legs?
                  ii.   Square window: How far can the baby's hand be flexed toward the wrist?
                  iii.   Arm recoil: How far can the baby's arms spring back to the flexed position?
                  iv.   Popliteal angle: How far can the baby's knees extend?
                  v.   Scarf sign: How far across his/her chest can the baby's elbows be moved?
                  vi.   Heel to ear: How close can the baby's feet be moved to his/her ears?
      c.   Gestational age determined based upon the sum of scores
                  i.   Low scores indicate immaturity
                  ii.   High scores indicate mature or post mature infant

Vital Signs

Variant to activity level

1.   Temperature: > 100.4°F (38°C) considered fever
2.   Pulse: 120 to 170 beats per minute (bpm)
3.   Respiration: 30 to as high as 80 breaths per minute (BPM)
4.   Blood pressure: < 112/74 mmHg

Skin

1.   Typical color changes: Pallor, cyanosis, plethora, jaundice, grey
2.   Milia: Pinpoint white papules on face, prominent on cheeks, nose, chin, and forehead
      a.   Spontaneously disappears within 3 to 4 weeks of life
      b.   If persist or wide spread distribution, especially if seen with other associated defects, may indicate trichodysplasia or oral-facial-digital syndrome type 1
3.   Miliaria: Obstructed sweat (eccrine gland) ducts; sometimes referred to as "prickly heat"
4.   Transient neonatal pustular melanosis: Vesicopustules
5.   Erythema toxicum: Most common newborn rash; usually appears between day 2 to 5 after birth; characterized by blotchy red spots on the skin with overlying white or yellow papules or pustules; resolves by the 14th day
6.   Cafe au lait spots: Typically a subtle shade discoloration located on either flank; may not be present at birth but likely to increase in size with age; suspect neurofibromatosis if there are many large spots or if > 6 spots in a child < 5 years of age
7.   Junctional nevi: If present in large numbers, suspect tuberous sclerosis, xeroderma pigmentosus, or generalized neurofibromatosis

8. Additional skin variations:
   a. Mongolian spots: Benign, flat, congenital birthmark with wavy borders and irregular shape; common color is blue; may last up to 3 to 5 years after birth, almost always by the puberty
   b. Port wine stain: Vascular birthmark (malformation) consisting of superficial and deep dilated capillaries in the skin; produce a reddish to purplish discoloration of the skin; permanent
   c. Hemangiomas: Benign, self-involuting vascular tumors that usually appear during the first weeks of life and resolve by age 10
   d. Strawberry marks: Affects 2% or more of babies; raised, soft red lumps on the skin, more common in premature babies; hypo/hyper-pigmented; after 6 months of age, the strawberry marks usually begin to shrink and fade

Neurological Exam

1. Level of consciousness, alertness
2. Posture: Hips should be abducted and partially flexed with knees flexed, arms adducted, elbows flexed, and fists clenched
3. Tone: Head should stay in line for 3 seconds
4. Reflexes should be symmetrical; survival reflexes: sucking and rooting

Reflex	Appears	Disappears
Rooting	Newborn	3 to 4 months
Sucking	Newborn	3 to 4 months
Moro	Newborn	3 to 4 months
Grasp (Palmar; Plantar)	Newborn	3 to 6 months; 4 months
Placing/stepping	Birth	1 to 2 months
Tonic Neck	Newborn	3 months
Babinski	Newborn	12 months or when walking
Reflex	Appears	Disappears

Head/Neck

1. Head shape/size variations
   a. Caput succedaneum: Crosses midline (fluid swelling); resolves in 2 to 3 days
   b. Cephalohematoma: Does not cross midline (blood); 5 to 10% up to 25% have an underlying fracture
   c. Bossing: Rickets, prematurity
   d. Microcephaly: Head circumference smaller than 2 standard deviations (SD); small brain

e. Macrocephaly: Head circumference larger than 2 SD, hydrocephalus, increased intracranial pressure (ICP)

f. Overriding sutures

2. Hair patterns and hair growth

    a. Color should match race

    b. Be uniform in color and distribution

    c. White forelocks with other anomalies are sometimes associated with deafness and retardation (Waardenburg syndrome)

    d. Hairline should not exceed the lower ear pole at the nape of neck; also assess for hair growth:

        i. More than one hair whorl could mean poor brain growth

        ii. Unruly hair with unusual facies, SGA, and microcephaly are found in Down syndrome

3. Fontanels

    a. Anterior fontanel is the largest (2 to 5 cm); closes by ~ 18 months

    b. Posterior fontanel may not be palpable at birth; closed by 2 to 3 months

    c. Common causes of wide fontanels

        i. Prematurity

        ii. IUGR

        iii. Hydrocephalus

        iv. Down Syndrome

        v. Hypothyroidism

        vi. Rickets

4. Eyes

    a. Colobomas (embryonic fissure defect): Mild forms only affect the iris; in more severe cases, the choroid and optic nerve can be involved with suspicion for central nervous system (CNS) midline defects such as optic nerve hypoplasia

    b. Heterochromia

    c. Cloudy cornea

    d. Red reflex

        i. Red reflex replaced by a black spot means there is no clear pathway from the lens to the retina

        ii. If replaced by a whitish color, this may suggest retinoblastoma or congenital cataracts; the sclera is normally white and may appear bluish in premies; if the sclera is deep blue, osteogenesis imperfecta should be ruled out

        iii. Salt-and-pepper speckling (Brushfield spots of the iris) is associated with Down syndrome

5. Ear/Nose/Throat Assessment

    a. Ear symmetry, pits, skin tags

       b.   Choanal atresia (narrowing or blockage of the nasal airway by tissue, present at birth)

       c.   Mouth/palate: Size/shape

       d.   Macro/microstomia, fish mouth

           i.   Microstomia (small mouth) is observed in trisomy 18 and 21

           ii.   Macrostomia (large mouth) is present in mucopolysaccharidoses; fish mouth is seen in fetal alcohol syndrome

       e.   Cleft lip/palate

       f.   Tongue

           i.   Macroglossia: Due to hypothyroidism, mucopolysaccharidoses

       g.   Teeth

           i.   Epstein pearls

           ii.   Natal teeth

6.   Chin: Micognathia in Pierre-Robin syndrome, Treacher-Collins syndrome, Hallerman Streiff syndrome

7.   Neck: Clavicular fractures, web neck, lymph nodes

Pulmonary

1.   Respiratory rate/pattern

       a.   Chest: Abdominal breathers

2.   Retractions

3.   Stridor

4.   Grunting

5.   Breast Enlargement

Cardiovascular

1.   Capillary refill

2.   Radio-femoral pulse delay: Consider coarctation

3.   Character of pulses

4.   Note the location and size of the point of maximum impulse (PMI): 3rd to 4th intercostal space (ICS)/left midclavicular line (LMCL)

5.   Murmurs: 85% of newborns have murmurs

Abdomen

1.   Contour: Flat abdomen is abnormal

2.   Gastroschisis

3.   Omphalocele

4.   Umbilical cord/number of vessels (2 arteries and 1 vein)/color

5.   Palpation of abdominal organs: Assess

6.   Hernias

7.   Anal patency

8.   Diastasis recti (rectus abdominis muscle separation)

Genitourinary

1.   Palpate kidneys: 4 to 5 cm
2.   Male genitalia
      a.   Penis: 3.5 to 4 cm stretched
            i.   Inspect glans, urethral meatus (hypo/epispadias)
            ii.   Inspect circumcised penis for edema
            iii.   Note ability to retract foreskin in uncircumcised penis
      b.   Note presence of testes: 97% of full term males have descended testes at birth
3.   Female genitalia
      a.   Discharge/small amount of bleeding may be present

Musculoskeletal

1.   Spine
      a.   Scoliosis
      b.   Kyphosis
      c.   Lordosis
      d.   Spinal defects
      e.   Meningomyeloceles
2.   Clavicular fracture
3.   Fingers/creases
4.   Developmental dysplasia of the hip (DDH): With hips flexed at 90 degrees and knees together, begin by abducting, then adduct while the examiner's fingers are over the greater trochanters
      a.   Ortolani's sign: A "click" is heard or felt
      b.   Barlow's maneuver: Feeling of a slip as the femoral head slips away from the acetabulum

The Newborn Assessment: Selected Screening Tests

Screening Considerations

1.   Be sure to screen for disorders in which symptoms would not be clinically present until irreversible damage occurs
2.   Screen for disorders for which there is a cure
3.   Consider the prevalence of a disease in the population
4.   Use of a simple screening method
5.   Screening has low false positive/false negative results
6.   High benefit-to-cost ratio
7.   There is a mechanism for follow-up after diagnosis

Mandatory Screening Program

1.   Established more than 30 years ago

2. Goal: Early identification of specific metabolic disorders
3. All 50 states require: Phenylketonuria (PKU), galactosemia, sickle cell disease, congenital hypothyroidism
4. Tests available for over 50 conditions

Considerations for Newborn Screening

1. A re-screen is mandatory for newborns tested at < 24 hours of age
2. Re-screen infants who appear symptomatic
3. Premature infants may have a low T4 indicating hypothyroidism
4. Sensory Conditions
   a. Vision Screening
      i. Identify risk factors for visual problems
         1. Prenatal infection
         2. Perinatal infection
         3. Congenital cyanotic heart diseases (hyperoxygenation)
         4. Structural malformations
         5. Family history of vision problems
         6. Hyperoxygenation in the neonatal period
         7. Absent red reflexes
   b. Hearing screening
      i. Observe response to loud noise/voice (startle reflex)
      ii. Brain stem auditory evoked response (BAER) test: Auditory brain stem response
      iii. Evoked otoacoustic emissions
      iv. Should be identified at birth but no later than 3 months and treated by 6 months
5. Inborn errors of metabolism
   a. PKU
      i. Occurrence: 1:10,000 to 25,000
      ii. Developmental delay
      iii. Severe retardation
      iv. Seizures
      v. Aggression
      vi. Autism
      vii. Hyperactivity
   b. Galactosemia: Liver dysfunction, coagulopathies
      i. Occurrence: 1:60,000 to 80,000
      ii. Special Consideration: 25% of unrecognized infants develop sepsis
         1. Organism usually *E. coli*
         2. Sepsis by 1 to 2 weeks of life
   c. Maple syrup urine disease

       i.   Tested in at least 23 states
       ii.   Occurrence: 1:250,000 to 300,000
       iii.   Ketoacidosis
       iv.   Mental retardation
       v.   Neurological impairment
       vi.   Death within the first 2 weeks of life is not uncommon

6. Hemoglobinopathies
   a.   Sickle cell disease
       i.   Occurrence: 1:400 African Americans
       ii.   Anemia
           1.   Thalassemia is also tested in some states
       iii.   Sepsis
       iv.   Vaso-occlusive crisis
       v.   Osteomyelitis

7. Endocrine-related Disorders
   a.   Hypothyroidism
       i.   Occurrence: 1:3,600 to 5,000
       ii.   Mental retardation
       iii.   Neurologic abnormalities
       iv.   Metabolic abnormalities
       v.   Special consideration: Presents with a late onset in 10% of cases
   b.   Congenital adrenal hyperplasia
       i.   Ambiguous genitalia
       ii.   Salt losing crisis
       iii.   Milder forms may occur

8. Miscellaneous conditions
   a.   Cystic fibrosis: Pulmonary disease, pancreatic insufficiency, cirrhosis, failure to thrive (FTT); has range of severity
   b.   Homocystinuria
       i.   Mental retardation
       ii.   Marfanoid body
       iii.   Dislocation of eye lenses
       iv.   Osteoporosis
       v.   Thromboembolic disease
   c.   Biotinidase deficiency
       i.   Alopecia
       ii.   Skin rashes
       iii.   Developmental delay
       iv.   Hypotonia
       v.   Ataxia
       vi.   Hearing/vision abnormalities
   d.   Toxoplasmosis
       i.   Obstructive hydrocephalus

        ii.   Chorioretinitis
        iii.   Intracranial calcification
        iv.   Severe infection may cause cardiopulmonary or nephrotic problems

e.   Tyrosinemia
        i.   Failure to thrive
        ii.   Hemolytic anemia
        iii.   Fanconi syndrome

Sample Questions

1.   Which of the following is the most accurate description of the Dubowitz tool?

   a.   It evaluates the physical condition of the newborn at birth.
   b.   The criteria evaluated are influenced by labor and birth; therefore, a second exam may be indicated to pick up any changes in the newborn.
   c.   It is a gestational assessment tool that evaluates the infant's newborn reflexes including the Moro reflex, tonic neck, grasping, rooting, and sucking.
   d.   Estimations of gestational age are performed by examining physical characteristics and neuromuscular development of the newborn.

2.   A full-term newborn had a birth weight below the 10th percentile, with length and height in the 50th percentile. The maternal history was positive for anemia, preeclampsia, and two prior miscarriages. What is the most likely diagnosis?

   a.   Intrauterine growth retardation (IUGR) secondary to chronic hypertension
   b.   Anemia secondary to maternal deficiency
   c.   Small for gestational age secondary to chromosomal abnormalities
   d.   Asymmetric IUGR

3.   Which of the following is the most accurate statement regarding newborn screening?

   a.   Sickle cell disease and cystic fibrosis screening tests are required in all 50 states.
   b.   Screening is performed for disorders in which there is no cure.
   c.   Screening is performed using a simple screening method.
   d.   Phenylketonuria (PKU), glactesemia, and hypothyroidism screening tests are performed in all symptomatic newborns.

Answers

1. Correct Answer: D
The APGAR evaluates the physical condition of the newborn at birth. Labor and the birth process do not affect the Dubowitz. The Dubowitz is a gestational assessment tool, but it evaluates both neuromuscular and physical maturity and is not based on newborn reflexes.

2. Correct Answer: D
The newborn has asymmetric IUGR, most likely secondary to pre-eclampsia. Chronic hypertension usually causes symmetric IUGR, where the height, weight and head circumference are all below the 10th percentile. A newborn with anemia would show other symptoms. Severe maternal malnutrition can cause symmetrical IUGR. There is not enough data to support the suspicion of chromosomal abnormalities.

3. Correct Answer: C
Sickle cell disease screening is mandatory in all 50 states but cystic fibrosis screening is not. Screening is performed when there is a cure. Screening is performed using simple screening methods. PKU, glactesemia, and hypothyroidism are all mandatory screening tests that are performed on all newborns, not just those that are symptomatic.

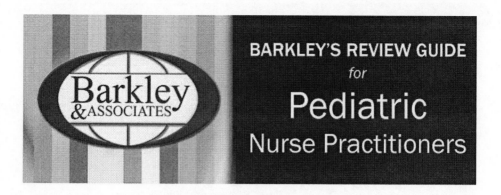

Growth and Development

The Domains of Growth and Development

Growth and development is a phrase used to describe the multifaceted process of development of the whole person. Three primary domains (Physical, Cognitive, and Psychosocial) are typically described, each of which are comprised of multiple factors. Disturbances among any of these factors may, theoretically, alter growth and development. Optimal growth and development ideally requires universal, domain development. In reality, the experience of human growth and development is not ideal, and the unique characteristics of the individual are a result of imbalances, excess and deficits among the fundamental domains.

The Physical Domain

Physical growth occurs in an orderly, predictable sequence influenced by individual variability.

Individual Variability

1.   Inherited genetic characteristics (e.g., height, weight)
        a.   Growth deviations could be "constitutional"
                i.   Large head (benign familial megalencephaly)
                ii.   Small head can sometimes be familial, but more frequently associated with developmental delay
        b.   A greater number of males experience constitutional growth delay with delay in the onset of puberty
        c.   Sequential measurements important
2.   Congenital syndromes/malformations
3.   Ethnicity
4.   Cultural practices

Nutritional Factors

1.   Caloric requirements vary according to age
        a.   Birth to 6 months: 110 to 120 kcal/kg/day
        b.   5 months to 1 year: 95 to 100 kcal/kg/day
        c.   1 to 3 years: 102 kcal/kg/day
        d.   4 to 6 years: 90 kcal/kg/day

e. 7 to 10 years: 70 kcal/kg/day
f. Adolescence
   i. Males
      1. 11 to 14 years: 55 kcal/kg/day
      2. 15 to 18 years: 45 kcal/kg/day
   ii. Females
      1. 11 to 14 years: 47 kcal/kg/day
      2. 15 to 18 years: 40 kcal/kg/day

Breast vs. Bottle:

1. Breast feeding
  a. Is the perfect food for humans; cannot be duplicated
  b. Good synchrony with breathing
  c. Decreases illness in infant
    i. Immunoglobulin isotype (IgA) [not normally acquired until 4 months of age; blocks influenzae and streptococcus from attaching to respiratory epithelial cells (50% less otitis media)]
    ii. Maternal antibodies are transferred to infants
  d. Decreased gastrointestinal problems such as gastroesophageal reflux diease (GERD)
    i. Breast milk is protective against diarrheal illness
    ii. Breast milk considered clear liquid and digested quicker that formula; therefore, continue through gastric distress
  e. Decreases allergies as breast milk contains anti-inflammatory agents to decrease atopy (fewer allergies in children who are breastfed)
  f. Breastfeeding during painful procedures provides analgesia
  g. The longer the mother breastfeeds, the less chance of the child to be overweight independent of education and socioeconomic status
  h. Economic reasons: Formula costs approximately $1,200/year

Exclusive breast feeding for 6 months

1. Feed on demand
  a. Adequate nutrition confirmed by weight gain
    i. 30 g/day (1 oz/day) for the first 3 months
    ii. Gain of 15 to 20 g/day during subsequent 3 months
  b. Vitamin Supplementation
    i. Supplementation with most vitamins controversial
    ii. Vitamin D supplements [200 International Units (IU) per day] at 2 months of age to adolescence
    iii. Vitamin B12 for breastfeeding mothers who are strict vegetarians (neurological abnormalities)

    c.   Iron
        i.   For exclusively breast-fed infants: Approximately 1 mg/kg/day of iron is recommended after 6 months of age
        ii.   Bottle feeding should contain iron supplementation
        iii.   Ideally, the iron should come from fortified cereals
        iv.   Elemental iron supplements can be given if iron intake from diet not adequate

    d.   Fluoride supplements only when local water supply is deficient
        i.   Supplementation is not needed for the first 6 months of life
        ii.   If drinking water supply has < 0.6 parts per million (ppm) of fluoride, begin supplementation
            1.   6 months to 3 years: 0.25 mg per day
            2.   3 to 6 years: 0.5 mg per day
            3.   6 to 16 years: 1 mg per day
        iii.   If drinking water supply has 0.3 to 0.6 ppm of fluoride
            1.   Birth to 3 years: None
            2.   3 to 6 years: 0.25 mg per day
            3.   6 to 16 years: 0.5 mg per day
        iv.   If drinking water has more than 0.6 ppm of fluoride, no supplemental fluoride is necessary

Weight gain progression

1.   Rapid decelerating growth followed by consistent growth
    a.   Initial 10% loss
    b.   Regained within 7 to 14 days
    c.   Doubles by 5 months of age
    d.   Triples by 1 year of age
    e.   Quadruples by 2 years of age
2.   Absolute vitamin, mineral and water requirements are substantially less in infancy; progress with age/weight

Catch-up growth requirements for malnourished infants and children

1.   Catch-up energy needs (kcal/kg/day) =

$$\frac{\text{RDA* calories for age} \times 50^{th} \text{ percentile weight for height (kg)}}{\text{Actual weight (kg)}}$$

2.   Determine the child's required caloric intake per day (use above values)
3.   Determine the child's weight (at the 50th percentile) for child's height (ideal body weight for height)
4.   Multiply the required calories by the ideal body weight

---

* Recommended dietary allowance

5.   Divide this value by the child's actual weight

Tooth Eruption

1.   Mandibular, then Maxillary, Incisors, Cuspids, Molars (Come Little Children Munch Meat)

Primary Teeth	Age of Eruption in Months
Central Incisor	6 to 7.5
Lateral Incisor	7 to 9
Cuspid	16 to 18
First Molar	12 to 14
Second Molar	20 to 24
Permanent Teeth	Age of Eruption in Years
Central Incisor	6 to 8
Lateral Incisor	7 to 9
Cuspid	9 to 12
First Bicuspid	10 to 12
Second Bicuspid	10 to 12
First Molar	6 to 7
Second Molar	11 to 13

The Cognitive Domain

Information Processing

1.   Encompasses receipt and processing of environmental stimuli
2.   Development begins in the newborn
3.   Initially, development centers around the ability to receive environmental input
    a.   Vision
    b.   Hearing
    c.   Reflexes
4.   A variety of principles are used to describe cognitive development from infancy through adolescence: Predominate theory is Piaget's Theory of Cognitive Development
    a.   Reflexes
    b.   Egocentrism, animism
    c.   Invincibility
    d.   Exaggerated sense of importance

Communication
1.   Receptive ability precedes expressive
2.   Responds to sounds at birth
3.   Ability to respond to increasingly complex language
4.   Development of abstract thought abilities

Cognitive and Psychosocial Domain

Development from Individual to Environmental
1.   Development of temperament
2.   Parent infant interaction
3.   Attachments
4.   Fears
5.   Home environment
6.   Social environment
7.   Play
8.   Aggression/impulse control
9.   Gender identity
10.   Interpersonal relationships/intimacy
11.   Goals

Psychosocial Development Theories
1.   Sigmund Freud
2.   Erik Erikson
3.   Jean Piaget
4.   Carl Roger

Major Theories of Growth and Development

There are numerous theories of growth and development along the physical, cognitive, psychosocial, and moral domain.

Jean Piaget

Theory of Cognitive Development
1.   Sensorimotor stage: Birth to 2 years
        a.   Reflexes: Inborn
        b.   Adapts inborn reflexes to the environment
        c.   Object permanence
        d.   Sensory abilities improve; becomes increasingly aware of environment
        e.   Trial and error learning
        f.   Simple problem-solving
2.   Preoperational (preconceptual) thinking: 2 to 7 years
        a.   Can focus on a single aspect of a situation

       b.   No cause-and-effect reasoning
       c.   Egocentrism
       d.   Development of intuitive thought
       e.   Difficulty distinguishing fact from fantasy (magical thinking)

3. Preoperational (intuitive) thinking: 4 to 7 years
   a. Beginning of causation
4. Concrete thinking: 7 to 11 years
   a. Capable of logical thought
   b. Logical operations
5. Formal operational thought: 11 to 15 years
   a. Ability to abstract
   b. Capable of complex problem solving
   c. Reality-based

Erik Erikson

Characterized by major tasks or stages across the lifespan

1. Infancy (birth to 1 year): Trust v. mistrust
2. Toddler (1 to 3 years): Autonomy v. shame and doubt
3. Preschool (3 to 6 years): Initiative v. guilt
4. School age (6 to 12 years): Industry v. inferiority
5. Adolescence (12 to 18 years): Identity v. role confusion
6. Successful psychosocial development requires successful resolutions of these developmental tasks

Sigmund Freud

Theory of Psychosexual Development

1. Three components or personalities are developed (or not) by experiences in particular stages of development
   a. Id: Principle of pleasure
   b. Ego: Principle of reality/self-interest
   c. Superego: Principle of morality or conscience
2. Stages of psychosexual development
   a. Infancy: Oral stage
   b. Birth to 6 months: Orally passive (development of the id; biological pleasure principle)
   c. 7 to 18 months: Orally aggressive (teething); oral satisfaction of needs by mother decreases tension
   d. Toddler (1.5 to 3 years): Anal stage
   e. Preschool (3 to 6 years): Phallic stage (love of opposite sex, Oedipal complex); ego development
   f. School age (6 to 12 years): Latency stage (sexual drive repressed, socialization occurs, super ego and morality development)

   g. Adolescence (12 to 18 years): Genital stage
3. Individuals can reduce anxiety and conflict by the use of defense mechanisms; these mechanisms are mental devices that distort reality to diminish psychic pain
  a. Repression
  b. Regression
  c. Sublimation
  d. Reaction formation
  e. Denial
  f. Rationalization

Other Theories

Bonding (Klaus & Kennel) and Attachment (Bowlby) Theories

1. Applies the principles of ethology to human beings
2. Attachment is viewed as being similar to imprinting
3. Intimate contact between mother and infant during the first few hours after birth is important in the development of an emotional bond with the baby
4. Attachment is necessary for infants to survive
5. According to Bowlby, infant attachments during the first 6 months of life are broad
6. After 6 months, attachment becomes more specific

Sensitive Periods of Development (Hinde)

1. There are sensitive periods for development of language, emotional attachment, and social relationships
2. Any deficit during these sensitive periods may have an adverse effect on the child; much depends on how severe the early deprivation and which later environmental influences meet important needs

Nurture Theories: Emphasizes Learning and Environment

1. John Watson: Classic conditioning
2. B.F. Skinner: Mechanistic-learning theory
3. Robert Bandura: Social learning theory

Humanistic Theory

1. Abraham Maslow: Theory centers around basic needs (hierarchy of needs) and human potential
2. Carl Rogers: Client-centered approach

Transactional Theories

1. Heredity: Environment
2. Transactional perspective

Growth and Development Landmarks

Individual stages of growth and development with a comprehensive outline of landmarks follows in subsequent sections

1.   Assessment of landmarks should be determined using corrected age for premature infants; this is especially true when performing the Denver Developmental Screening Test, second edition (Denver II) assessment

Calculating Corrected Age			
Step 1:	Calculate child's age in months:		
	Year	Month	Day
	2011	09	21 (today's date)
−	2010	06	03 (birth date)
	1	03	18 chronological age to 16 mos.
Step 2:	Determine # of weeks child was born early:		
	40 weeks = term		
−	27 weeks = gestational age		
	13 weeks = # of weeks born early		

Assessment of Developmental Tasks

Normally occurs in stages whereby development at one stage has an effect on the development of subsequent stages:

1.   Physical tasks
2.   Cognitive tasks
3.   Psychosocial tasks

Measurement Tools for Growth and Development Landmarks

Growth Parameters

1.   Growth charts
2.   Norms expressed as percentile of height, weight, head circumference for age
3.   Sequential measurements
4.   Any child who crosses over multiple sequential percentile lines needs further evaluation
5.   Body mass index (BMI) should be calculated and plotted for children over 2 years old
6.   BMI = $\dfrac{\text{(Weight in kg)}}{\text{(Height in meters)}^2}$
7.   Bone age: X-ray of tarsals and carpals determines extent of ossification

Cognitive Development
1.   Measurement by various standardized intelligence tests (IQ)
2.   Need at least 2 separate test results to make an assessment of intellect
3.   Can use toys and language-based assessment based on mental age

Denver II
1.   Generalized assessment tool
2.   Used from birth to 6 years of age
3.   Measures:
       a.   Gross motor development
       b.   Fine motor development
       c.   Language
       d.   Personal-social development
4.   Not an intelligence test
5.   Correct age for premature infants

See charts regarding **Growth and Development Milestones** and **Milestones by Age** on pages 26 and 27 respectively.

Growth and Development Milestones

Gross Motor	Months	Fine Motor	Months	Language	Months
Good head control	2–3	Grasps and shakes rattle	2–3	Smiles and coos	2–3
Rolls back to front	5–6	Reaches for object	3–4	Laughs	4–5
Sits alone	5–6	Hand-to-hand transfer	5–6	Babbles	5–6
Pulls to stand	9–10	Raking grasp	6–7	"Mama-Dada"	8–9
Stands alone	11–12	Finger grasp	7–9	Waves bye-bye	8–9
Walks	12–14	Pincer grasp	8–10	Understands "No"	9–10
Walks up and down stairs	22–24	Marks on paper	10–12	Points to body parts	15–18
Jumps	24–28	Stacks 3 blocks	17–18	3-word sentences	18–22
		Stacks 6 to 7 blocks	22–24	30-to-50-word vocabulary	22–24

Milestones by Age

2 to 5 months	Smiles and coos
	Watches a person's face intently
	Follows people and objects with eyes
	Laughs aloud
	Lifts head/chest when on stomach
	Holds head steady when pulled to sit
	Grasps rattle placed in hand
	Startles to loud noise
6 to 9 months	Babbles and combines vowel/consonant sounds
	Turns to sound
	Responds to name
	Rolls over
	Sits independently
	Transfers objects
	Supports weight on feet
	Uses thumb and fingers to pick up objects
	Crawls
10 to 12 months	Takes simple action upon request
	Purposefully says "Mama" or "Dada"
	Sits independently and plays
	Pulls to standing/cruise furniture
	Communicates by reaching and pointing
	Moves purposefully to get desired object
	Has increasing curiosity
	Recognizes people
	Uses both hands equally well
13 to 18 months	Scribbles with large crayon
	Walks alone
	Feeds self with fingers and begins using a spoon
	4 to 10-word vocabulary
	Follows simple directions
	Coordinates use of both hands
	Responds to name
	Points to 2 pictures upon request
	Long jabbering sentences
	Throw ball overhead
19 to 24 months	Walks up/down stairs
	Jumps with both feet
	Completes simple puzzles, circle shapes first
	Stacks 6 to 7 blocks
	Uses 2-word sentences
	30-to-50-word vocabulary

Sample Questions

1. You are examining a 6-month-old who has been fussy and drooling more often lately. The mother thinks the child is teething and has questions regarding tooth eruption. Which of the following is most accurate regarding tooth eruption in children?

   a. The lateral incisor is usually the first tooth to erupt.
   b. The first tooth eruption usually occurs at age 6 months.
   c. The primary teeth are usually all in by 18 months of age.
   d. Tooth eruption occurs in random order.

2. The new mother of a 2-month-old brings her baby to your office for a well child visit. The mother is considering switching from breast milk to formula because she is worried that she is not producing enough milk. Which of the following is the most appropriate response?

   a. Remind the mother that formula is more expensive than breast milk
   b. Inform her that breast milk is easier to digest and decreases allergies and illness in the infant
   c. Discuss and demonstrate the growth of the baby on the growth chart
   d. Advise the mother to follow the American Academy of Pediatrics recommendations and continue breastfeeding

3. You are seeing a well child. Currently, the baby can release objects, as well as grasp them, and use both arms together to manipulate. He chews on things, rather than merely mouthing them, and is able to grasp and examine his feet. When held upright just above the ground, he begins to show a walking reflex. He can also react to threatening presences such as strangers. His vocalizations are babblings with primitive speech. His age based on the description would be:

   a. 2 months
   b. 4 months
   c. 6 months
   d. 8 months

Answers

1. Correct Answer: B

The central incisor and lateral incisor are the first to erupt at age 6 to 7.5 months and 7 to 9 months, respectively. The primary teeth are not complete until age 24 months. Teeth erupt in an orderly fashion: Incisors, followed by cuspids, then molars.

2. Correct Answer: C

All of the answers are good reasons to breastfeed, but the mother is concerned that she is not making enough milk. Demonstrating the baby's growth on the growth curve should help her make this decision. Although the American Academy of Pediatrics recommends breastfeeding, the role of the PNP is to provide the relevant facts and allow parents to make the final decision.

3. Correct Answer: C

All of the behaviors listed are indicative of a 6-month-old child.

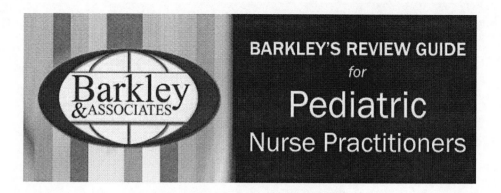

Infant Health Considerations

Child Health Supervision

A strategy designed to promote health and positive developmental outcomes

1. Routine health supervision is composed of systematic, comprehensive measures that not only promote health and development but also reduce morbidity and mortality by way of a proactive screening approach
2. Components of Child Health Supervision include health promotion strategies, specific screenings at regularly scheduled intervals, and implementation of anticipatory guidance
3. The American Academy of Pediatrics' (AAP) *Bright Futures: Guidelines of Health Supervision of Infants, Children, and Adolescents* serves as a primary guide for child health supervision

Definition

1. Newborn period: 1 to 2 months
2. Infancy: 1 to 12 months

Focus

1. Physical: Gross motor (cephalocaudal) and fine motor (proximal > distal) development
2. Cognitive: Sensorimotor
3. Psychosocial: Developing trust

Well Child Checks (WCC)

According to the *Bright Futures* guidelines, the schedule for an infant from ages 2 weeks to 1 year is at 2 weeks, followed by 2, 4, 6, 9, and 12 months.

If discharged from hospital prior to 48 hours, first visit should be within 3 to 5 days.

1. Schedule: Subjective data
   a. Feeding
   b. Elimination
   c. Sleep
   d. Development

      e.   Parental/caregiver concerns

      f.   Interval history: Health since last visit, emergencies, illness, medications

2.   Objective data

      a.   Length, weight, head circumference percentage, vital signs

      b.   Caregiver/infant interaction

      c.   Vision/hearing screening

      d.   Physical examination

      e.   Developmental screening [Denver Developmental Screening Test, second edition (Denver II) or equivalent]

      f.   Laboratory

          i.   Bilirubin if indicated

          ii.   Hematocrit between 6, 9, and 12 months, unless otherwise indicated

3.   Plan of care

      a.   Immunizations: Initiation of primary series

      b.   Illness management with medications

      c.   Health promotion strategies with anticipatory guidance

Specific Tools of Infant Health Screening

1.   Parent/caregiver interview
2.   Physical examination
3.   Developmental monitoring
4.   Specific, stage-appropriate screenings
5.   Assessment of strengths/weaknesses
6.   Individualized and evidence-based interventions

The Interview

General Approach

1.   Ascertain who will be present
2.   Ensure privacy
3.   Inform parents ahead of time if you are recording data
4.   Keep child clothed until necessary to remove clothing
5.   Phrase your questions purposefully
6.   Convey interest/listening
7.   Employ cultural sensitivity
8.   Ensure accurate perception of parents' concerns
9.   Use a non-judgmental approach

The Physical Examination: Necessary Elements

1.   Length
2.   Weight
3.   Head circumference (up to 2 years)

4. Serial measurements recorded with standardized charting
5. Dental development
    a. Central incisors
    b. Lateral incisors
    c. Cuspids
    d. First molars
6. Vital signs
    a. Pulse
        i. Newborns: 120 to 170 beats per minute (bpm)
        ii. At 1 year: 80 to 160 bpm
        iii. At 2 years: 80 to 140 bpm
    b. Respiration
        i. Newborns: 30 to as high as 80 breaths per minute (BPM)
        ii. By age 2: 20 to 30 BPM
    c. Blood pressure not routinely measured until 3 years of age
7. Head size, shape, fontanels
8. Head control by 4 months
9. No lag when pulled to sitting at 6 months; lag may be first sign of palsy
10. Assess for neck masses
11. Close inspection of head for evidence of syndromes previously presented
12. Skin variations
13. Assess for periorbital edema
14. Flattened or flaring nose
15. Nasal discharge
16. Mouth/throat exam: History may indicate abnormalities
    a. Too little/too much fluoride
    b. Sleeping with bottle
    c. Unusual tooth eruption sequence
    d. Fissures at lip corners: Vitamin deficiency
    e. Asymmetrical enlarged tonsil: May suggest tonsilar lymphoma
17. Voice
    a. Nasal/voice quality
    b. Shrill, high pitch: Increased intracranial pressure (ICP)
18. Heart sounds
    a. Point of maximum impulse (PMI): 4th intercostal space (ICS), midclavicular line (MCL)
    b. Innocent murmurs
    c. Always systolic
    d. Grade I or II
    e. Loudest when recumbent or after exercise
    f. No thrill
    g. Pulmonic ejection murmur
    h. Still's murmur
    i. Venous hum

19. Chest/lung exam
    a. Diaphragmatic breathers
    b. Pectus carinatum (pigeon chest)
    c. Pectus excavatum (sunken chest; the most common congenital deformity of the anterior wall of the chest)
    d. Gynecomastia/galactorrhea up to 3 months of age
20. Abdomen
    a. Prominent abdomen
    b. Liver edge palpable 1 to 2 cm below right costal margin
    c. Diastasis recti (separation of the rectus abdominis muscle)
21. Labial adhesions
22. Phimosis (unable to fully retract foreskin)
23. Testes fully descended by 3 months of age
24. Large scrotum
25. Genitourinary (GU) abnormalities such as hypospadius
26. Musculoskeletal
    a. Barlow's and Ortolani's tests for developmental dysplasia of the hips
    b. Allis's sign: Unequal leg length
    c. Scoliosis: Visual curvature
    d. Galeazzi's sign: Unequal knee height
    e. Skin fold thickness asymmetry
27. Lymph nodes
    a. 1 cm inguinal, 2 cm cervical enlargement (palpable) may be a normal variant
    b. Shotty nodes indicate past infection
    c. Supraclavicular nodes require aggressive investigation

Developmental Monitoring

Standardized Tests

1. Newborn Behavioral Assessment Scale (NBAS)
2. Bayley Infant Neurodevelopmental Screener (BINS)
3. Bayley Scales of Infant Development (BSID-II)
4. Ages and Stages Questionnaire (ASQ)
5. Denver II

Reflexes and Motor Skills

1. Assessment of reflexes
    a. Survival reflexes
        i. Breathing
        ii. Temperature control
        iii. Feeding
    b. Non-survival reflexes

          i.   Babinski: Movement of the big toe toward the top of the foot and other toes outward after the sole of the foot has been firmly stroked

          ii.   Stepping

          iii.   Moro: Awareness of falling sensation as demonstrated by a startled reaction

          iv.   Grasping

2. Gross motor skills
   a. Head control: 4 months
   b. Front to back roll: 4 to 5 months
   c. Back to front roll: 5 to 6 months
   d. Sits alone: 5 to 6 months
   e. Creeps/crawls: 7 to 9 months
   f. Pulls to stand/cruises: 9 to 10 months
   g. Stands alone: 12 months
   h. Walks forward: 12 to 14 months
3. Fine motor skills
   a. Grasp/shake rattle: 2 to 3 months
   b. Reaches for object: 3 to 4 months
   c. Hand to hand transfer: 5 to 6 months
   d. Unilateral reaching: 6 months
   e. Raking grasp: 6 to 7 months
   f. Finger feed: 7 to 9 months
   g. Pincer grasp: 8 to 10 months
   h. Marks on paper: 10 to 12 months
   i. Opens book/turn page: 12 to 13 months
   j. Stacks two blocks: 12 to 15 months

Cognitive Development

1. Blink reflex and pupil constriction indicate newborn vision
2. Newborns focus up to 30 inches
3. Binocular vision by 6 months
4. Visual acuity: Assess response to environment, voice
5. Hearing: High risk infants need screening
   a. Detects loss of 20 to 30 decibel hearing level (dB HL)
   b. Infants have greater acuity for high pitch
6. Sensori-motor development
   a. Adaptation of reflexes to environment
   b. Simple problem-solving without trial and error
7. Language development
   a. Smiles/coos: Age 2 to 3 months
   b. Laugh: 4 to 5 months
   c. Dada/mama: 8 to 9 months
   d. Waves bye-bye: 8 to 9 months

      e.   Understands "no": 9 to 10 months

      f.   Words other than mama/dada: 11 to 12 months

Psychosocial Development

1. Differentiation of temperament
   a. Easy
   b. Slow-to-warm
   c. Difficult/cyclic
2. Development of fears
   a. Strangers: By 6 months
   b. Separation: By 8 months
3. Attachment: Affective bond that develops over the first year and will differentiate into other emotions later
   a. Secure
   b. Insecure (detachment issues)
      i. Insecure: Avoidant
      ii. Insecure: Anxious
      iii. Insecure: Disorganized

Stage Appropriate Screenings

In Infancy

1. Hearing/screening as noted (AAP goal: Identify hearing loss before 3 months; treat by 6 months)
2. Tuberculosis (TB) screening: Not universal, based upon risk
3. Hematocrit at 6, 9, and 12 months

Anticipatory Guidance

Nutrition/Feeding

1. Breast feeding and bottle feeding
2. When to introduce other foods
3. Supplements
4. Nutritional requirements
5. Avoid common allergens
6. Weaning

Dental Health

1. Baby bottle tooth decay
2. Fluoride
3. Brushing
4. Cleaning schedule (first dental visit by 1 year of age)

Injury Prevention

1. Car seats

2.   Poison control numbers
3.   If more than 30 minutes to a healthcare facility (e.g. rural area), Ipecac
      may be used as directed by a Poison Control Center
4.   Electrical exposure protection
5.   All poisons out of reach
6.   Gates to barricade unsafe areas
7.   Smoke/carbon monoxide detectors
8.   Pool safety
9.   Crib safety
10.   Hot water safety
11.   Sun safety

Sleep

1.   Two months to 1 year: 8 to 12 hours per night
2.   Two to 3 naps daily
3.   Avoid sleeping with infant
4.   After night feedings end, do not pick up the baby during the night

Other Preventive Measures

1.   Passive/secondary smoke
2.   Potential for abuse/neglect
3.   Domestic violence
4.   Sexual abuse
5.   Firearms

Developmental Discussion/Guidance

1.   How to perform simple tasks
2.   When to call a health care provider
3.   Expected responses to immunizations and procedures
4.   Time management
5.   Discipline

Developmental Warning Signs

1.   Apparent visual delay
2.   Does not raise head when lying on stomach by 3 months
3.   Does not try to pick up a toy by 6 months
4.   No reactions to noise/voice
5.   Does not laugh
6.   Does not seek interpersonal contact
7.   Does not sit up

Sample Questions

1. Developmental monitoring in infancy involves observing infant milestones. Which physical characteristics are important to observe during physical development of the infant?

    a. Head circumference, length, weight, vision, and teething
    b. Head circumference, length, weight, vision, and toilet training
    c. Length, weight, vision, vocalization, and toilet training
    d. Head circumference, length, weight, vision, and vocalization

2. You are examining a smiling and cooing baby who grabs the stethoscope from your neck with one hand and transfers it to her other hand. The best assessment of the baby's age is:

    a. 2 to 3 months
    b. 3 to 4 months
    c. 4 to 5 months
    d. 5 to 6 months

3. The provider is taking a history from a new patient who is 8 months old. When asking about day care, the mother explains that the infant has been attending day care since age 2 months, but lately she screams as if she has never been there before and clings to her mother when she is left in the mornings. What is the provider's best information for the mother concerning this behavior?

    a. Something must be wrong in the environment and mother should consider another option for care.
    b. The mother needs to spend more time with her baby to ascertain attachment.
    c. The infant is displaying separation anxiety, and this is normal.
    d. Socializing the infant with strangers will alleviate this fear.

Answers

1. Correct Answer: A

These infant development stages are perhaps the easiest of all the infant milestones to track. There are 5 characteristics that are important in physical development. These five criteria are: head circumference, length, weight, vision, and teething.

2. Correct Answer: D

The infant's fine motor skills develop in a consecutive order with grasp and rattle-shaking starting at 2 to 3 months, reaching for object at 3 to 4 months, hand-to-hand transfer at 5 to 6 months, and unilateral reaching at 6 months.

3. Correct Answer: C

At certain stages, most babies or toddlers will show true anxiety and be upset at the prospect (or reality) of being separated from a parent. However, separation anxiety will pass, and there are ways to make it more manageable. The development of fears in babies is normal and often displays as fear of strangers by 6 months and fear of separation by 8 months.

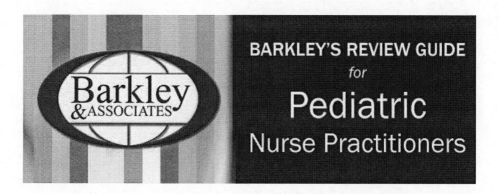

Toddler and Preschool Health Considerations

Definition
1. Toddler: 1 to 3 years of age
2. Preschool: 4 through 5 years of age

Periodicity Guidelines

Stage Appropriate Screenings
1. Schedule:
   a. Toddler: 12, 15, 18, and 24 months
   b. Preschooler: Annually at 3, 4, and 5 years
2. Subjective data: Same as infant (see "Well Child Checks" on page 31)
   a. Nutrition
   b. Elimination
   c. Sleep
   d. Development
   e. Parental and caregiver concerns
   f. Interval history: Track health since last visit including emergencies, illness and/or medications
3. Objective data: Similar to the infant with some anthropometric and lab differences
   a. Anthropometrics:
      i. Toddler: Length, height, weight, head circumference percentage (up to 2 years old)
      ii. Preschooler: Height, weight, blood pressure (starting at 3 years old, then each year)
   b. Caregiver/child interaction and parenting style
   c. Vision and hearing screening
   d. Physical exam
   e. Developmental screening [Denver Developmental Screening Test, second edition (Denver II) or equivalent]
   f. Laboratory:
      i. Toddler:
         1. Urinalysis at 2 years unless otherwise indicated

        2.   Hematocrit at 2 years (or once between 1 and 5 years unless otherwise indicated)

        3.   Lead screening (questionnaires) by 2 years as appropriate based on well child surveillance of risk (for more information, see the guidelines outlined by the Centers for Disease Control on page 237)

    ii.   Preschooler

        1.   Purified protein derivative (PPD) test for tuberculosis between 4 and 6 years if at risk

        2.   Cholesterol screening around 2 years; test if indicated (e.g., family history, dyslipidemia or premature cardiovascular disease)

4.   Plan of care:

    a.   Immunizations

    b.   Illness management with medications

    c.   Health promotion strategies with anticipatory guidance

    d.   Dental screening; first screening at least by age 3

    e.   American Academy of Pediatrics (APA) currently recommends first screen at 1 year

Specific Tools of Child Health Screening

1.   Parent and caregiver interview
2.   Physical examination
3.   Developmental monitoring
4.   Specific, stage-appropriate screenings
5.   Assessment of strengths and weaknesses
6.   Individualized and evidence-based interventions

The Interview

General Approach

1.   Ascertain who will be present
2.   Ensure privacy
3.   Inform parents ahead of time if you are recording data
4.   Keep child clothed until necessary to remove clothing
5.   Talk to child at eye level
6.   Play to enhance comfort
7.   Use projective techniques
8.   Use non-threatening words
9.   Allow adequate time for response
10.   Seek necessary details

The Physical Examination

Maximize the interview

1. Toddler is striving for autonomy
2. Tantrums are common
3. Major fears emerge
4. Allow child to touch equipment
5. Give choices when possible
6. Continue progression of non-invasive to invasive exam
7. Minimum time undressed

Necessary Elements

1. Length: Each visit to 2 years, then annually to age 5
2. Weight: Each visit to 2 years, then annually to age 5
3. Head circumference is measured on each visit to 2 years of age
4. Serial measurements recorded with standardized charting
5. Dental development is by 3 years unless high risk progression
    a. Cuspids
    b. First molars
    c. Second molars
6. Vital signs
    a. Pulse: ~ 80 to 130 beats per minute (bpm)
        i. Pulse pressure should be 20 to 50 mmHg
        ii. Varied pulse pressures result from increased systolic pressure due to fever, exercise and excitation
        iii. Decreased diastolic pressure
    b. Respiration: As high as 20 to 40 breaths per minute (BPM)
    c. Blood pressure: ≤ 112/76 mmHg
        i. Blood pressure is taken beginning at age 3
7. Anterior fontanel closed by 18 months
8. Chest and head are equal to age 1; chest eventually grows 5 cm > head
9. Eye exam should be investigated
    a. Excessive squinting
    b. Difficulty picking up small objects
    c. Head tilting
    d. Strabismus
10. Tympanic membrane may be red due to crying
11. Assess for neck masses as swollen or shotty nodes may be normal
12. Mouth breathers: Cause may result from allergic rhinitis
13. Assess for periorbital edema
14. Nasal discharge
15. Mouth and throat exam is time to discontinue bottle use
    a. Too little or too much fluoride
    b. Unusual tooth eruption sequence

        c.   Fissures at lip corners indicate a vitamin deficiency

16.   Voice
        a.   Nasal quality including adenoids
        b.   Raspy voice can be from multiple causes

17.   Cardiac
        a.   Increased respiration rate during sleep
        b.   Eyelid edema
        c.   Squatting or sleeping in knee-to-chest position
        d.   Exercise intolerance
        e.   Heart sounds
            i.   Point of maximal impulse (PMI) near the 4th intercostal space (ICS) or midclavicular line (MCL)
        f.   Innocent murmurs
            i.   Always systolic
            ii.   Grade I or II
            iii.   Loudest when recumbent or after exercise
            iv.   No thrill
        g.   Pulmonic ejection murmur heard in the pulmonic area, early to mid-systole; distinct gap between first heart sound and murmur and end of murmur and second heart sound
        h.   Vibratory or Still's murmur is a musical or vibratory murmur; heard best at the lower left sternal border
        i.   Venous hum is heard best above or below clavicles; second or third ICS may note more coarse quality and is position dependent; can disappear with lying down or turning of neck

18.   Chest/lung exam
        a.   Assess for family history of lung disease or hypersensitivity
        b.   Sudden onset of cough

19.   Abdomen
        a.   Prominent abdomen
        b.   Liver edge palpable 1 to 2 cm below the right costal margin
        c.   Diastasis recti: A separation between the left and right side of the rectus abdominis muscle

20.   Labial adhesions
21.   Phimosis: A condition in which the foreskin is tightly stretched around the head of the penis and cannot be pulled back freely
22.   Undescended testes
23.   Musculoskeletal
        a.   Genu varum (bow legs) normal in toddlerhood
        b.   Genu valgum (knock-knees) normal in preschooler
        c.   Turned in foot
24.   Femoral anteversion
25.   Tibial torsion
26.   Lymph nodes

     a.   One centimeter inguinal; two centimeter enlargement may be normal variant in the inguinal or cervical region

     b.   Supraclavicular nodes require aggressive investigation

Developmental Monitoring

Motor Skills

1.   Gross motor skills
   - a.   Walks forward at 12 to 14 months
   - b.   Walks backward at 14 to 16 months
   - c.   Walks up steps at 16 to 18 months
   - d.   Walks up/down steps alone at 20 to 24 months
   - e.   Two foot jump at 20 to 24 months
   - f.   At 2 years:
     - i.   Up and down steps
     - ii.   Kicks ball without falling
     - iii.   Runs with wide gait
   - g.   At 3 years:
     - i.   Hops at 3.5 years
     - ii.   Rides a tricycle
   - h.   At 4 years:
     - i.   Up and downs stairs with alternating feet
     - ii.   Rides bicycle with training wheels
   - i.   At 5 years:
     - i.   Skips
     - ii.   Jumps rope
     - iii.   Plays ball

2.   Fine motor skills
   - a.   Uses utensils at 15 to 17 months
   - b.   Stacks 3 blocks at 17 to 18 months
   - c.   Simple puzzles at 18 to 20 months
   - d.   Stacks 6 or7 blocks at 20 to 24 months
   - e.   At 2 years
     - i.   Tower of 8 cubes
     - ii.   Turns a doorknob
   - f.   At 3 years
     - i.   Copies a circle
     - ii.   Builds a tower
   - g.   At 4 years
     - i.   Draw person with 4 to 6 parts
     - ii.   Tower of 10 blocks
   - h.   At 5 years
     - i.   Copies a square
     - ii.   Copies multiple shapes

        iii.   Prints letters
        iv.   Ties shoes

Cognitive Development

1. Piaget's preoperational thinking stages
   a. Preconceptual occurs at age 2 to 4 years
   b. Intuitive begins at age 2 to 7 years
   c. Centration occurs as focus is on one thing at a time
   d. Egocentrism: The tendency of children to cognize their environment only in terms of their own point of view
   e. Animism begins, projecting the ability to think/feel like the child, inanimate objects are capable of feeling/thinking
2. Visual acuity to 20/30 by 5 years
   a. Snellen chart
   b. Tumbling E
   c. HOTV eye chart test
   d. Allen card
   e. Broken Wheel
   f. LH symbol test
3. Hearing
   a. Orientation to sound and language development begins at 2 years
   b. Two to 3 years, play audiometry
   c. Over 3 years, should experience pure tone audiometry
4. Language development
   a. By age 2:
      i. Up to a 50-word vocabulary
      ii. Can follow two-step commands
      iii. Talks constantly
   b. By age 3:
      i. Up to a 900-word vocabulary
   c. By age 4:
      i. Can understand phrases and simple analogies
   d. By age 5:
      i. Vocabulary > 2000 words
      ii. Uses sentences
      iii. Knows at least 4 colors

Psychosocial Development

1. Autonomy vs. shame and doubt (developing sense of self)
2. Introduction of discipline
3. Aggression and impulse control
4. Play is a major psychosocial medium
   a. Toddlers: Onlooker and parallel play
   b. Preschoolers: Associative, cooperative, dramatic, physical

Stage Appropriate Screenings

Office Visits

1. Hearing/screening as noted
2. Blood pressure each year; begin age 3
3. Cholesterol count at 2 years especially if family history of dyslipidemia or premature cardio vascular disease
4. Lead poisoning questionnaires to determine those at high risk
5. Routine urine screening at 2 years
6. Hematocrit once at age 1 to 5 years
7. Dental screening with first screening occurring at least by age 3
8. The AAP recommends the first screen at 1 year

Standardized Testing

1. Bayley scale for infant development, second edition (BSID-II): Goal standard for the diagnosis of developmental delays in infants to 42 months of age; separate mental, motor and behavioral rating scales
2. Ages and stages questionnaire (ASQ)
3. Denver II
4. First Step
5. McCarthy Scales of Children's Abilities
6. Weschler Preschool and Primary Scale of Intelligence Revised
7. Early Language Milestone Scale
8. Receptive and Expressive Emergent Language Scale
9. MacArthur Communicative Development Inventories
10. Toddler Temperament Scale

Anticipatory Guidance

Nutrition/Feeding

1. Off the bottle and drinking from cup
2. Encourage use of utensils
3. Avoid simple sugar snacks and drinks
4. Do not force eating

Dental Health

1. Brushing after meals and before bed
2. First dental exam by age 3 (or by 12 months for high-risk children)

Injury Prevention

1. Car seats
2. Poison control numbers
3. Ipecac: Make available in certain situations; if > 30 minutes to a health care facility or as directed by a poison control center
4. Electrical exposure protection

5. All poisons out of reach
6. Gates and barricades are unsafe areas
7. Smoke/carbon monoxide detectors
8. Pool safety
9. Crib safety
10. Hot water safety
11. Sun safety

Sleep

1. Sleeps 10 to 12 hours per night with daily naps
2. Rituals and consistency at bedtime
3. Nightmares begin around age 3
4. Night terrors occur between 2 to 4 years if child does not wake up

Toilet Training

1. Physiologic and psychologic readiness begins between 1.5 and 2.5 years
2. Average daytime control is achieved by 24 months
3. Nighttime control lags behind by 1 year compared to daytime control
4. Do not start in times of stress
5. Do not punish
6. Reward all good efforts
7. Limit time on the potty

Other Preventive Measures

1. Avoid passive and secondary smoke
2. Watch for abuse/neglect potential
3. Watch for domestic violence
4. Watch for sexual abuse
5. Lock up firearms

Developmental Discussion/Guidance

1. How to perform simple tasks
2. When to call a health care provider
3. Expected responses to immunizations and procedures
4. Time management
5. Discipline
6. As child develops language skills, encourage parents to listen/respond

Developmental Warning Signs

1. At 1 year:
   a. Is not imitating sounds
   b. Is not pulling to standing
   c. Is not indicating desires by point/gesture
2. At 18 months:

        a.   Does not make eye contact
        b.   Does not feed self with spoon
        c.   Does not squat spontaneously

3.   At 2 years:
        a.   Is not walking up stairs
        b.   Is not using 2-to-3-word phrases
        c.   Is not noticing cars, animals
        d.   Is not initiating self-stimulation behaviors

4.   At 3 years:
        a.   Is not aware of external environment
        b.   Cannot ride a tricycle
        c.   Does not follow simple direction
        d.   Continues baby talk
        e.   Does not imitate adult activities

5.   At 4 years:
        a.   Does not listen to a story
        b.   Does not speak in sentences
        c.   Engages in head banging or rocking
        d.   Is not toilet trained
        e.   Does not draw a human figure

6.   At 5 years:
        a.   Magical thinking is still a dominant presence
        b.   There is no impulse control

Sample Questions

1. The predominant characteristic of the intellectual development of the child age 2 to 7 years is egocentricity. Which of the following best describes this concept?

   a. Selfishness
   b. Self-centeredness
   c. Prefers to play alone
   d. Unable to put self in another's place

2. Which of the following is characteristic in the development of a 2½-year-old child?

   a. Birth weight has doubled.
   b. Primary dentition is complete.
   c. Anterior fontanel is open.
   d. Binocularity may be established.

3. In the clinic waiting room, a nurse observes a parent showing an 18-month-old child how to make a tower out of blocks. The nurse should recognize which of the following in this situation?

   a. Blocks at this age are used primarily for throwing.
   b. Toddlers are too young to imitate the behavior of others.
   c. Toddlers are capable of building a tower of blocks.
   d. Toddlers are too young to build a tower of blocks.

Answers

1. Correct Answer: D

Jean Piaget (1896-1980) claimed that young children are egocentric. This does not mean that they are selfish but that they do not have the mental ability to understand that other people may have different opinions and beliefs. Their tendency to perceive, understand and interpret the world in terms of the self.

2. Correct Answer: B

Birth weight doubles by 3 to 4 years. While the posterior and lateral fontanels are obliterated by about 6 months after birth, the anterior is not completely closed until about the middle of the second year. It is normal in the first 6 months for a baby's eyes to become crossed occasionally, but by one year binocularity (using both eyes together) develops, and the eyes will then work as a pair. Primary dentition is the best answer and is complete by around 2 years of age.

3. Correct Answer: C

Fine motor development during toddlerhood consists of refinements in reaching, grasping, and manipulating. The 18-month-old can make a tower of blocks. One year later, he can stack eight blocks. Most 18-month-olds will hold the crayon in a fist and scribble spontaneously.

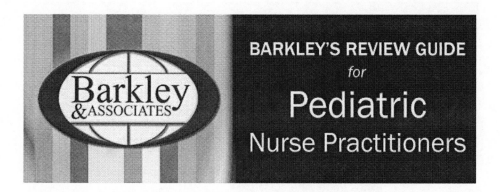

BARKLEY'S REVIEW GUIDE
for
Pediatric
Nurse Practitioners

School Age Health Considerations

Definition

School age: 6 through 12 years of age

Focus

Physical

1.   Latency period (Sigmund Freud's stages of psychosocial development)
2.   Growth of 2.5 inches/year
3.   Growth of 5 to 7 lbs per year

Cognitive

1.   Conceptual

Psychosocial

1.   Industry stage (Erik Erikson's stages of psychological development)
2.   Desire to please adult figures

Well Child Checks (WCC)

Bright Futures/Periodicity Guidelines

Annual Stage Appropriate Screenings

1.   Elimination (constipation, enuresis)
2.   Development (school, activities, exercise, friends, behavior, family relationships)
3.   Risk factors/behaviors (alcohol, tobacco and other drugs, especially caffeine for older children)

Physical Examination

1.   Body mass index (BMI)
2.   Scoliosis
3.   Tanner Staging

Laboratory

1. Purified protein derivative (PPD) test for tuberculosis once before school entry at 4 to 6 years of age
2. Annually if any of the following risk factors are present:
    a. Low socioeconomic status
    b. Residence in areas where tuberculosis is prevalent
    c. Exposure to tuberculosis
    d. Immigrant status
    e. Hematocrit (typically once) at 8 years; additional as needed
    f. Cholesterol if family history dyslipidemia or premature cardiac disease

Management Plan

1. Immunizations [2nd vaccine against measles, mumps and rubella (MMR) for school entry]
2. Illness management with medication
3. Health promotion strategies with anticipatory guidance
4. Dental assessment and cleanings every 6 months

Well Child Check Notable Points

The Interview

General Approach

1. Ascertain who will be present
2. Ensure privacy
3. May use diagrams (visuals are best)
4. Interview while fully-clothed

Maximize the Interview

1. Industry vs. inferiority
2. Child wants to be brave
3. Older school age children become more modest
4. Fears pain, loss of control, death

The Physical Examination: Necessary Elements

1. Rapid physical growth and development levels off (latent period)
    a. Average 10 year old is 70 lbs. and 52 to 56 inches tall
        i. Average growth: 5 to 7 lbs/year; 2 to 3 in/year
    b. Girls reach peak height velocity (PHV) at age 11 to 12 (prior to menarche)
    c. Height, weight and BMI
        i. If BMI is between the 85th and 95th percentiles, the patient is at risk for becoming overweight

        ii.   A BMI above the 95th percentile indicates obesity

2.   Vital signs each visit (pulse and respiration rate decrease; blood pressure increases)
      a.   Pulse: 75 to 115 beats per minute (bpm)
      b.   Respiration: 16 to 20 breaths per minute (BPM)
      c.   Blood pressure: < 126/82 mmHg
3.   Physical exam proceeds from head to foot
4.   Visual acuity approaches 20/20
5.   Permanent teeth erupt
6.   Girls become thoracic breathers
7.   Breast development begins in girls
8.   Scoliosis screening beginning age 9: Curves > 30% may need bracing

Developmental Monitoring

Motor Skills

1.   Motor skills are well developed
2.   Muscle strength increases
3.   Hand dominance emerges

Cognitive Development

Erikson's industry vs. inferiority stage: Child is active, energetic, and curious

1.   Jean Piaget's concrete operational thinking stage
2.   Cognitive tasks at this age are varied and include
      a.   Acquiring new knowledge and sense of industry
      b.   Thought processes expand: Is capable of reversibility
      c.   Can grasp the concept of conservation
      d.   Can classify things based upon one characteristic
      e.   Language becomes fluid and descriptive
      f.   Can use concepts of time and money
      g.   Masters cause and effect
      h.   Understands concept of space
      i.   Capable of deductive reasoning

Psychosocial Development

1.   Marked expansion to include the outside world
2.   Development of self-esteem
      a.   Feels competent in abilities: Learning, decision-making, etc.
      b.   Believes he/she is worthy of love
3.   Socialization
      a.   Plays with others, organized sports
      b.   Interested in peer groups, clubs
      c.   Capable of behaving in a peer environment
      d.   Toward late school age, peers become extremely important

4.   Responsibility
    a.   Will be proactive to meet needs
    b.   Can fulfill household and school responsibilities
    c.   Will often seek moneymaking opportunities with limited responsibility (such as babysitting, dog-walking, etc.)

Anticipatory Guidance

Unique to age group

Nutrition/Feeding

1.   Institution of the food guide pyramid
2.   Minimize "junk" food
3.   May appear to have increased weight as linear growth stabilizes (average gain annually: 2.5 inches)

Dental Health

1.   Brushing after meals and before bed
2.   Dental cleaning every 6 months
3.   Placement of sealants
4.   Learn how to floss

Injury Prevention

1.   Seat belts
2.   Poison control numbers
3.   Electrical exposure protection
4.   All poisons out of reach
5.   Make ipecac syrup available in certain situations; if > 30 minutes to a healthcare facility such as in rural setting or as directed by a Poison Control Center
6.   Smoke/carbon monoxide detectors
7.   Pool safety
8.   Hot water safety
9.   Sun safety
10. Helmets while riding bicycles, roller skating
11. Teach pedestrian safety
12. How to use 911
13. Stranger safety

Sleep

1.   Sleep 8 to 10 hours per night
2.   Nightmares decrease

Sexuality

1.   Increased curiosity about opposite sex
2.   Establish communication about sexually-transmitted infections (STIs), human immunodeficiency virus/acquired immune deficiency syndrome (HIV/AIDS)
3.   Prepare girls for menstruation, males for hormonal/body changes
4.   Give accurate information about sexual intercourse; reinforcement over time is vital

Other Preventive Measures

1.   Communication about cigarette, drug, alcohol abuse
2.   Passive/secondary smoke
3.   Abuse/neglect potential
4.   Domestic violence
5.   Sexual abuse
6.   Firearms

Developmental Discussion/Guidance

1.   Discipline
    a.   Consistency is critical
    b.   Adults must role model
    c.   Should emphasize natural and logical consequences
    d.   Should be assigned regular duties/chores
    e.   As child develops language skills, encourage parents to listen/respond
2.   Reinforce honesty
3.   Respect need for privacy
4.   Be aware of television programming and internet activity (should be < 2 hours/day)
5.   Expect lying: Confront child in a positive way

Developmental Warning Signs

1.   In younger school age children:
    a.   Poor adjustment to school
    b.   Not working to ability
    c.   Frequent illnesses/need to stay home from school
    d.   Lack of social interaction/peer problems
2.   In older school age children:
    a.   Revert to dependent, shy, passive roles
    b.   Using illness to avoid responsibilities
    c.   Cannot make or keep friends
    d.   Poor school performance (feeling "left behind")
    e.   Disinterest in any extra academic activity

f.   Destructive behavior to express self

Sample Questions

1. Which of the following statements accurately describes physical development during the school-age years?

   a. The average child's weight triples.
   b. The average child grows an average of 2 inches per year.
   c. Most children are thin at this age due to "picky" eating.
   d. Fat gradually increases, which contributes to a child's heavier appearance.

2. Which of the following describes the cognitive abilities of school-age children?

   a. They have developed the ability to reason abstractly.
   b. They become capable of scientific reasoning and formal logic
   c. They progress from making judgments based on what they reason to making judgments based on what they see.
   d. They have the ability to classify, to group and sort, and to hold concepts in their minds while making decisions.

3. A father tells you that he is concerned about his 12-year-old son getting "fat." His son is at the 50th percentile for height and the 75th percentile for weight on the growth chart. What is the most appropriate action to take?

   a. Reassure the father that his son is not "fat"
   b. Reassure the father that his son is just a growing child
   c. Suggest a low-calorie, low-fat diet
   d. Explain that this is typical of the growth pattern of boys at this age

Answers

1. Correct Answer: B

Two inches per year is the average growth of a child. However, no child grows at a perfectly steady rate throughout this period of childhood. Weeks or months of slightly slower growth alternate with mini "growth spurts" in normal children. A major growth spurt occurs at the time of puberty. Girls usually enter puberty between ages 8 and 13 years, and boys between 10 and 15.

2. Correct Answer: D

School age children begin to classify in terms of hierarchical relationships (e.g., both fish and birds are animals). They explore objects visually rather than manually. Most first and second grade children have the capacity for abstract thinking as long as it pertains to something they have directly experienced. They are able to make comparisons with their own experiences. Although they learn best through concrete experiences, they can utilize books as an additional source of information. While these children have a deepening ability to distinguish between fantasy and reality, they enjoy pretending and acting out stories.

3. Correct Answer: D

Using a pediatric growth chart, one would see that this child is within normal limits. To use the chart, find the child's age along the bottom and draw a straight line going up, parallel to the right and left sides of the chart. Then find the child's height along the side and draw a line across, marking the point where the child's age line and height line cross. By looking at the boys' growth chart, you can tell that a 10-year-old boy who is 55 inches tall is of average size (50th percentile) for his age. A 10-year-old boy who is only 50 inches tall, however, falls at about the 5th percentile.

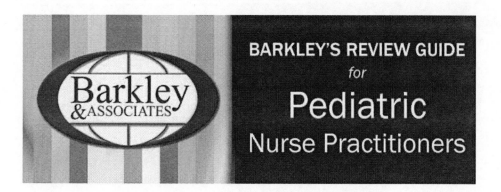

Adolescent Health Considerations

Definition

1. Adolescence: 12 through 20 years of age
2. Bridging from school age to adulthood
3. Three transitional periods:
   a. Early adolescence: 11 to 13 years
   b. Middle adolescence: 14 to 16 years
   c. Late adolescence: 17 to 20 years

Focus

Physical

1. Rapid changes in the reproductive, skeletal, muscular, and cardiovascular systems
2. Secondary sexual characteristics
3. Peak height velocity (PHV)

Cognitive

Logical, abstract thinking

Psychosocial

1. Sense of identity
2. Narcissism

Well Child Checks (WCC)

Bright Futures/Periodicity Guidelines: Annually

Stage Appropriate Screenings

1. Elimination (laxatives, diuretics)
2. Development
   a. Mental/emotional health
   b. School performance and attendance; friends and relationships
   c. Family functioning

       d.   Hobbies and activities

       e.   Work

       f.   Stress, anger management, and coping skills

       g.   Risk-taking behaviors

       h.   Injury to self or others

3.   Risk factors/behaviors

       a.   Alcohol, tobacco, drugs, or caffeine (especially for older children)

4.   Sexual activities and reproductive issues

5.   Concerns and worries: Current and recent stressors

6.   Specific questions to ask when alone with parents:

       a.   Family communication patterns and relationship

       b.   Description of adolescent's strong and weak points, attitudes, and behaviors

       c.   Discipline practices and responses

       d.   Specific concerns and worries about the adolescent

Physical Examination

1.   Observation of the parent/adolescent interactions

       a.   Is the parent supportive of the adolescent?

       b.   Does the parent allow the adolescent to answer questions?

2.   Body mass index (BMI)

3.   Physical examination including:

       a.   Assessment for scoliosis (until 2 years after PHV)

       b.   Tanner staging

       c.   Clinical breast exam

       d.   Pelvic exam (if sexually active, irregular menses, etc.)

       e.   Breast self-exam (BSE)

       f.   Testicular self-exam (TSE)

Laboratory

1.   Hematocrit as needed

2.   Syphilis test (VDRL), gonorrhea test (GC), chlamydia, and human immunodeficiency virus (HIV) if sexually active or history of sexual abuse

3.   Pap smear if pelvic exam is performed

4.   Liver function tests if history of drug usage

5.   Cholesterol if indicated

Management Plan

1.   Immunizations

       a.   Hepatitis B (HepB), especially for sexually active adolescents or those using drugs

       b.   Meningococcal vaccine

       c.   Diptheria, pertussis, and tetanus (DTaP)

       d.   Human Papillomavirus (HPV)

e. Measles, mumps, and rubella (MMR)
2. Illness management with medications
3. Health promotion strategies with anticipatory guidance
4. Dental assessment and cleanings every 6 months

Well Child Check Notable Points

Framework: Guidelines for Adolescent Preventive Services (GAPS) by the American Medical Association

The Interview

General Approach

1. Ensure privacy
2. May use diagrams and visuals
3. May need to structure part of the interview alone
4. Be alert for cues that the adolescent does not want to discuss certain issues in front of parents
5. Encourage expression of feelings and concerns
6. Interview while fully-clothed

Maximize the Interview

1. Adolescent is identity seeking
2. May be rebellious
3. Is often inflexible
4. Is refining sex role and sexuality
5. Trying to be independent

The Interview

General Approach

1. Strategy with the **HEAD** format
  a. **H**ome environment
  b. **E**mployment and education
  c. **A**ctivities
  d. **D**rugs
2. Strategy with the **PACES** format
  a. **P**arents, peers
  b. **A**ccident, alcohol/drugs
  c. **C**igarettes
  d. **E**motional issues
  e. **S**chool; sexuality
3. Strategy with the **SAFETEENS** format
  a. **S**exuality
  b. **A**ccident, abuse
  c. **F**irearms, homicide

    d.   **E**motions (suicide/depression)

    e.   **T**oxins (tobacco/alcohol, others)

    f.   **E**nvironment (school, home, friends)

    g.   **E**xercise

    h.   **N**utrition

    i.   **S**hots (immunization status and school performance)

The Physical Examination: Necessary Elements

1. Physical maturing: Secondary sexual characteristics developing; most significant physical changes are sexual
2. Vision and hearing screen at each visit
3. Vital signs each visit (more adult-like)
   a. Pulse: 60 to 100 beats per minute (bpm)
   b. Respiration: 16 to 20 breaths per minute (BPM)
   c. Blood pressure approaches adult norms
4. Physical exam proceeds from head to foot
5. Visual acuity: 20/20; may alter with hormone surging
6. Tanner staging
   a. Sexual maturity rating (SMR) is obtained by taking the average from both Tanner stage rates (genital + pubic hair development):
      i. Boys (secondary sexual characteristic development; penis and pubic hair development):
         1. Preadolescent testes, scrotum, penis
         2. Enlargement of scrotum and testes; scrotum roughens and reddens
         3. Penis elongates
         4. Penis enlarges in breadth and development of glans; rugae appear
         5. Adult shape and appearance
      ii. Girls (breast and pubic hair development):
         1. Preadolescent breasts
         2. Breast buds with areolar enlargement
         3. Breast enlargement without separate nipple contour
         4. Areola and nipple project as secondary mound
         5. Adult breast: Areola recedes, nipple retracts
      iii. Pubic hair (for both males and females):
         1. Preadolescent
         2. Sparse, pale, fine
         3. Darker, increased amount, curlier
         4. Adult in character but not as voluminous
         5. Adult pattern

Developmental Monitoring

Physical Development

1. PHV reached; associated with Tanner staging
2. Progresses from "long and gangly" to adult appearance (musculoskeletal development)
3. Females menstruate: Menarche between breast development stages 3 to 4; predominantly at stage 4
4. Males begin nocturnal emissions; spermarche occurs shortly after genital stage 3
5. Onset of puberty before age 8 in girls and 9 in boys is precocious puberty

Cognitive Development

1. Erikson's identity vs. role confusion stage
2. Piaget's abstract thinking stage
    a. Cognitive ability progresses to adulthood
    b. Younger adolescent daydreams; trouble staying focused
3. As adolescence progresses, becomes creative
4. Enjoys intellectual challenge
5. Uses humor and formal thought

Psychosocial Development

1. Younger adolescence
    a. Conforms to peer groups
    b. Characterized by parent/child conflict
    c. Expresses anger
2. Older adolescence
    a. Less emotionally labile
    b. Continues to develop independence
    c. Reestablishes rapport with parents
    d. More interested in opposite sex
    e. Better sense of self-esteem, confidence

Anticipatory Guidance

Nutrition/Feeding

1. Nutritional requirements are higher than adults
2. Minimize "junk food"
3. Encourage regular meals
4. Monitor vegetarian diets
5. Discuss dieting

Dental Health

1. Brushing after meals and before bed

65

2. Dental cleaning every 6 months
3. Teach flossing

Injury Prevention

1. Seat belts
2. Smoke/carbon monoxide detectors
3. Pool safety
4. Sun safety
5. Helmets while riding bicycles, roller skating
6. Teach pedestrian safety
7. Stranger safety
8. Discuss drug/alcohol use
9. Motor vehicle/driving safety (motor vehicle accidents are the #1 cause of death in this population)

Sexuality

1. Increased interest in the opposite sex
2. Establish communication about sexually-transmitted infections (STIs) and HIV/AIDS
3. Prepare for body changes, menstruation, or nocturnal emissions
4. Give accurate information about sex, disease prevention, and pregnancy prevention

Other Preventive Measures

1. Passive/secondary smoke
2. Abuse/neglect potential
3. Domestic violence
4. Sexual abuse
5. Firearms
6. Mental health (depression and/or suicide)
7. Gang activity

Developmental Discussion/Guidance

1. Discipline
   a. Negotiation is essential; allow some flexibility on less important issues
   b. Adults must be role models
2. Reinforce honesty
3. Respect need for privacy
4. Be aware of television programming and internet activity
5. Expect histrionics in young adolescents

Developmental Warning Signs

1. Change in school performance, friendships, sleeping, or eating

2. Apparent personality changes
3. Difficulty accepting failure
4. Talk of suicide
5. Withdrawal from friends or family

Sample Questions

1. Most female adolescents can be expected to begin menarche when:

   a. Pubic hair is sparse, pale, fine
   b. Areola and nipple project as a secondary mound
   c. Pubic hair is adult in appearance
   d. Breast buds appear with areolar enlargement

2. During the adolescent years, teens may see the provider irregularly. When teens come into the clinic, the provider should ascertain that they receive any immunizations that are normally given during adolescent. These would include:

   a. Hepatitis B (HepB), especially for sexually active adolescents or those using drugs, meningococcal meningitis, tetanus/diphtheria/pertussis vaccines (Tdap), human papillomavirus vaccine (HPV), and measles, mumps and rubella (MMR)
   b. Diphtheria/tetanus/pertussis vaccines (DTaP), MMR, and HepB
   c. HepB, especially for sexually active adolescents or those using drugs, meningococcal meningitis, and hib conjugate vaccine (Hib)
   d. MMR, HepB, and HIB

3. In accordance with adolescent interview guidelines, in the nurse practitioner office or clinical setting, you should always:

   a. Advise the adolescent that what they tell you may have to be confided to parents
   b. Hold the interview in a private setting and without parents
   c. Have parents and their teen in your office for conversation
   d. Have the adolescent fill out a questionnaire to save time

Answers

1. Correct Answer: B

Menarche typically begins between breast development stages 3 and 4, predominantly at stage 4, when areola and nipple project as a secondary mound.

2. Correct Answer: A

Hib is not given after age 5, and DTaP is not given after age 11. Tdap should be given at age 11 or 12 as a booster during the routine adolescent immunization visit.

3. Correct Answer: B

A part of any overall interview with an adolescent patient involves talking about alcohol and other drugs. This interview should be held in a private setting and without parents present. It is helpful to have related pamphlets prominently displayed, with multiple copies to give away. Pamphlets should include information about alcohol and drug use and other health related behaviors. Reassure the patient that your discussion is confidential and that you will not disclose the details of your conversation with parents without the patient's permission unless a serious health risk exists.

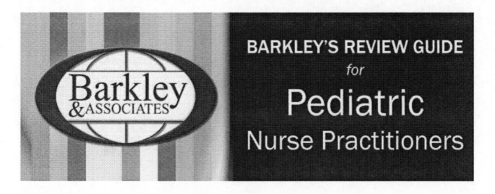
Immunization Recommendations

- The Advisory Committee on Immunization Practices (ACIP) publishes updated immunization schedules annually in January*
- Administration for all vaccines are typically 0.5 ml with the exception of the influenza vaccine

Hepatitis B Vaccination

Series of 3 from 0 to 6 months

1. All newborns: First dose before hospital discharge
1. First dose must be monovalent vaccine
2. In infants born to hepatitis B antigen (HBsAg) positive mothers:
   a. Administer hepatitis B vaccine (HepB) and 0.5mL hepatitis B immune globulin (HBIG) within 12 hours of birth
   b. Test for HBsAg and antibody to HBsAg after 3 or more doses of HepB series (at age 9 to 18 months)
3. If the mother's HBsAg status is unknown:
   a. Determine/check status immediately after birth
   b. Administer HepB within 12 hours of birth
   c. If mother tests positive, HBIG should be given no later than 1 week of age
4. Second dose: One to 2 months of age; monovalent or a combination vaccine containing HepB
5. Final dose should be given at 24 weeks of age or later, but not before 6 months of age

Rotavirus Vaccine (Rota)

Series of 3 from 6 weeks to 8 months

1. Administer first dose 6 to 14 weeks, and each subsequent dose at 4 week intervals

---

* For more information, see www.cdc.gov/vaccines/recs/acip

2. Must complete series before 32 weeks; do not administer a dose after the age of 32 weeks
3. *Note:* There is insufficient data on the safety and efficacy outside of these age ranges

Diphtheria/Tetanus/Pertussis Vaccines

Series of 3 primary and 2 boosters from 2 months to 6 years of age

1. First 3 doses given at 2, 4, and 6 months of age
2. First dose can be given as early as 6 weeks of age
3. Fourth dose can be given at 12 months if the provider suspects child will not return for 15 to 18 month vaccines
4. Fourth dose must be at least 6 months after third dose
5. Fifth dose is not necessary if the 4th dose was at age 4 years or more
6. Diptheria and tetanus toxoids vaccine (DT) is used in children less than 7 years old when the addition of pertussis is contraindicated
7. The preferred formulation for children less than 7 years old is the diphtheria, tetanus, and pertussis vaccine (DTaP)
8. DTaP is not indicated for children 7 years of age or older
9. Td vaccine is used in children 7 years of age or older
    a. Tetanus prophylaxis in wound management
        i. Depends on the nature of the wound
            1. Any open wound
            2. Wounds contaminated with dirt, feces, soil, or saliva
            3. Devitalized tissue (e.g., necrotic or gangrenous wounds)
        ii. Depends on the history of immunization with tetanus toxoid
            1. If history of last tetanus and diphtheria toxoids (Td) vaccination is unknown or the child received fewer than 3 doses prior to any type of wound:
                a. The child should receive a Td
                b. With any type of wound (other than a clean minor wound): The child should also receive tetanus immune globulin (TIG)
            2. Three or more doses of vaccine within the last 5 to 10 years with a wound (other than a clean minor wound): Give Td vaccine

3. Three or more doses of vaccine (with the last dose more than 10 years prior to any type of wound): Give Td vaccine

10. Administration: 0.5 mL intramuscularly

    a. The total number of DT and DTaP immunizations should not exceed 5 by the 4th birthday

Tetanus, Diphtheria, Acellular Pertussis Vaccines (Tdap)

Minimum age: 10 years for Boostrix and 11 years for Adacel

1. For those who have completed the recommended childhood DTP/DTaP vaccination series and:

    a. Have not received a Td booster: Administer at 11 to 12 years of age

    b. Are between the age of 13 to 18 but have missed the 11 to 12 year Td/Tdap booster: Administer a single dose of Tdap

2. Subsequent Td boosters are recommended every 10 years

Hib Conjugate Vaccine (Hib)

1. If haemophilus B conjugate [PRP-OMP (PedVax-Hib, ComVax)] is used at 2 and 4 months, no 6 month vaccine is required [2, 4, and 6 months optional; 12 to 15 months or older: a combination DTaP and haemophilus B conjugate vaccination (TriHIBit) – DTaP – Hib]

    a. Children without prior DTaP vaccine may have a better response to PRP-OMP than other formulations

2. First dose of Hib can be given as early as 6 weeks of age; not recommended for children 5 years of age or older

3. DTaP/Hib combination should not be used as primary Hib but can be used as a booster after initial vaccination with any Hib vaccine in children 12 month olds or older

4. Administration: 0.5 mL; intramuscularly

Pneumococcal Vaccine

PCV 7 or 23PS: Age dependent

1. Pneumococcal Conjugate Vaccine (PCV) 7 for all children younger than 23 months (23PS not approved for use in children younger than 2 years of age)

    a. 2 to 6 months of age: Primary series: 3 doses, 6 to 8 weeks apart (1 booster dose at 12 to 15 months of age)

    b. 7 to 11 months: Primary series of 2 doses, 6 to 8 weeks apart (1 booster dose at 12 to 15 months of age)

    c. 12 to 23 months of age: Primary series of 2 doses, 6 to 8 weeks apart

      d.   24 months or older: Primary series of 1 dose

2.   Children aged 24 to 59 months who received 4 doses of PCV 7 previously should receive the first dose of 23PS vaccine at 24 months of age (at least 6 to 8 weeks from last PCV 7) and second dose of 23PS at 3 to 5 years after the first dose of 23PS if they have the following:

      a.   Hemoglobinopathies
      b.   Asplenia
      c.   Splenic dysfunction
      d.   HIV infection
      e.   Congenital immunodeficiencies
      f.   Renal failure
      g.   Nephrotic syndrome
      h.   Chronic cardiac disease
      i.   Chronic pulmonary disease (except asthma)
      j.   Diabetes
      k.   Consider in this age group if of Native American, African American, or Alaskan descent, or attending day care

3.   Children aged 24 to 59 months with the above stated risk conditions for pneumococcal disease and have not been previously immunized with PCV 7 should:

      a.   Receive 2 doses of PCV 7 6 to 8 weeks apart
      b.   The first dose of 23PS vaccine, 6 to 8 weeks after the last dose of PCV 7
      c.   Second dose of 23PS vaccine 3 to 5 years after the first dose of 23PS

4.   Children aged 24 to 59 months with the above stated risk conditions for pneumococcal disease and have previously received 1 dose of 23PS should receive:

      a.   Two doses of PCV 7, 6 to 8 weeks apart, beginning at least 6 to 8 weeks from the initial 23PS vaccine
      b.   One dose of 23PS vaccine, 3 to 5 years after the first dose of 23PS vaccine was given

5.   PCV 7 indicated for:

      a.   Children older than 24 months at high risk for pneumococcal infection as described above

6.   Administration:

      a.   Dose of PCV 7: 0.5 mL; intramuscularly
      b.   Dose of 23PS: 0.5 mL; intramuscularly or subcutaneously

Polio Vaccine (IPV)

Series of 4 from 2 months to 6 years

1.   Inactivated polio vaccine (IPV) for all 4 in the series (from 2 months to 6 years of age)

2. First 2 doses given at 2 and 4 months of age
3. First dose can be given as early as 6 weeks of age
4. Third dose can be given between 6 and 18 months of age
5. Fourth dose is given between 4 and 6 years of age (before entry into school)
6. Oral polio vaccine (OPV) vaccine should be used only in the following situations:
   a. Mass vaccination to control outbreaks of paralytic polio
   b. Unimmunized children traveling (in less than 4 weeks) to areas where polio is endemic or epidemic
   c. Only for the third and/or 4th dose if a child's parents are opposed to the recommended number of injections to complete the polio immunization schedule

Influenza Vaccine (annually)

1. Administer annually to all children beginning at 6 months
2. In children 6 to 35 months of age, the dose = 0.25 mL intramuscularly; for children $\geq$ 3 years = 0.50 mL intramuscularly
   a. Whole or split virus is given to children older than 12; prior to this age only split virus given
   b. Live attenuated inactive virus (LAIV), known as FluMist, may be used as an alternative to trivalent inactivated virus (TIV) in healthy persons aged 2 to 49 years
   c. Split-virus vaccines are licensed for use in children older than six months of age
   d. Inactivated whole virus vaccines should not be used in children less than 13 years of age
3. First doses in children younger than 9 years should be divided into 2 administrations: 4 weeks or more apart for TIV, and 6 weeks or more for the LAIV

Measles, Mumps, and Rubella (MMR)

Two doses from 1 to 12 years of age

1. Second dose may be given as few as 4 weeks after the first
2. Both doses should be given after age 12 months and completed by 11 to 12 years [second dose routinely recommended for the 4 to 6 year well child check (WCC) visit; may be given at any age as many as 4 weeks apart]
3. If exposed to measles or travelling to endemic areas, can give MMR as early as 6 months of age, but the patient needs 2 additional doses (primary series) of vaccine at 12 to 15 months, and again at 4 to 6 years
4. Administration: 0.5 mL; subcutaneously
   a. May be given simultaneously with TB testing with purified protein derivative (PPD)

b.   If MMR given, postpone Purified Protein Derivative (PPD) for 4 to 6 weeks to avoid possible suppressive response of PPD

Varicella

Two dose series at minimum age of 12 months; may administer at any visit

1.   Give 2 doses after the age of 12 months when no reliable history of chicken pox and no evidence of immunity is available
   a.   Second dose is given at age 4 to 6 years
   b.   May administer prior to age 4 if it has been 3 months or more have elapsed since the first dose and both doses are given at age 12 months or older
   c.   Do not repeat second dose if administered 28 days or more following the first dose
2.   Administration
   a.   0.5 mL; subcutaneously
   b.   May give simultaneously with MMR, otherwise allow 1 month between MMR and varicella
   c.   Give 5 months after varicella zoster immune globulin (VZIG); do not give concurrently
   d.   Avoid salicylates for 6 weeks post vaccination to avoid neurological complications (Reyes syndrome)

Hepatitis A Vaccine

Series 2 two doses from 1 to 2 years of age

1.   Recommended for all children 12 to 23 months of age
2.   Administration:
   a.   Give two doses, the second dose given six months after the initial dose
   b.   If not fully vaccinated by the age of two, can be completed at subsequent visits
3.   Previous recommendations include:
   a.   Recommended in geographic regions in which incidence is twice the national average (consult local public health department)
   b.   Should be considered in geographic regions in which incidence exceeds national average
   c.   Highest incidence in children five to 14 years of age
   d.   Travelers
   e.   Men who have sex with men
   f.   Drug users
   g.   Clotting factor disorders
   h.   Chronic liver disease, including HBV or HCV
   i.   Attending day care *not* considered a risk factor

Meningococcal Vaccine
1.   Meningococcal conjugate vaccine [MCV4 (Menactra)]:
       a.   Recommended for all children ages 11 to 12
       b.   All previously unvaccinated children at high-school entry (around age 15)
       c.   All previously unvaccinated college freshmen living in dormitories
       d.   All others at high risk of invasive meningococcal disease and between the ages of 11 and 55

Human Papillomavirus Vaccine (HPV)

Series of 3 doses, females ages 11 to 12

1.   Two preparations commercially available, covering the oncologic strains of HPV
       a.   Human papilloma virus quadrivalent (types: 6, 11, 16 and 18) vaccine recombinant (Gardisil)
       b.   Human papilloma virus bivalent (types: 16 and 18) vaccine, recombinant (Cervarix)
2.   Indicated for ages 9 to 26 years (Gardisil) and 10 to 25 (Cervarix)
3.   Contraindicated in pregnancy

Catch-up Pearls
1.   Lapse in immunizations from recommended schedule: Resume immunizations according to schedule
2.   Repeat dosing is not indicated; no need to restart a vaccine series regardless of the time that has lapsed
3.   Pay attention to dosing intervals
4.   The immunization schedule for children younger than 7 years of age who have not received immunizations in the first year of life includes:
       a.   First visit: DTaP, Hib, HBV, MMR, IPV, PVC7/23PS, Rota, HepA
              i.   Hib and PCV7/23PS are not necessary if the child is 5 years of age or older and immunocompetent
              ii.   May combine DTaP and Hib after 15 months
              iii.   If age 2 to 7: May begin MCV4 series (for immunocompromised)
       b.   One month after the initial visit: DTaP, HBV, Var, Rota, Hib, MMR, IPV, PCV7/23PS
       c.   Two months after the initial visit: DTaP, Hib, IPV, PCV7/23PS, Rota
              i.   Second dose of Hib is necessary only if first dose given before 12 months
              ii.   Second dose of PCV7/23PS is indicated if the child is less than 2 years old
       d.   Eight months or more from the initial visit: DTaP, HBV, IPV, HepA

        i.   IPV and HBV are not necessary if the first three doses were given previously

    e.   4 to 6 years (at or before school entry): DTaP, IPV, MMR

        i.   DTaP is not necessary if the 4th dose is given after 4th birthday

        ii.   IPV is not necessary if third dose is given after 4th birthday

5.   Recommended immunization schedule for children 7 to 18 years old not immunized in the first year of life:

    a.   At first visit: HBV, MMR, Td/Tdap, IPV, HepA

        i.   For females ages 11 to 18: HPV (may be given as early as age 9)

        ii.   MCV4 series may be initiated (e.g., for immunocompromised patients, military recruits, and those living in a college dormitory)

    b.   Two months after initial vaccines: HBV, MMR, Var, Td/Tdap, IPV

    c.   Eight – 14 months after initial vaccines: HBV, Td/Tdap, IPV, HepA

        i.   IPV not needed at this visit if third dose was given earlier

        ii.   HBV not necessary at this visit if third dose given earlier

Common Adverse Responses

Hepatitis B

1. Adverse reactions are typically minor; local muscle soreness
2. There is no link of hepatitis B vaccine to multiple sclerosis

DTaP

1. None significant
2. Local erythema, tenderness
3. Low grade temperature
4. If boosters are given too often, arthrus (severe local pain and edema) may occur

Hib Vaccine

1. Local erythema, edema, warmth
2. Temperature to 101°F (38.3°C)

IPV

1. Local discomfort
2. Contraindicated in those with history of anaphylaxis to streptomycin

MMR

1. Local edema, induration
2. Low grade temperature
3. Mild rash

4. Joint pain may occur 1 to 3 weeks after vaccination
5. Adverse reactions due to the mumps live-virus vaccine is rare
   a. Orchitis and parotitis have been reported, but its occurrence is rare
   b. Other reactions that occur after immunization with MMR are attributed to the measles and rubella components of the vaccine
6. Should not be given to those who are pregnant or immunosuppressed
7. May be given to persons with HIV if CD4 cell/mm^3 more than 200
8. May be given to those with egg allergy; observe for 90 minutes postvaccination
9. No link between MMR and autism or inflammatory bowel disease

Varicella

1. Local tenderness
2. Erythema
3. Maculopapular or vesicular rash
4. Contraindicated in pregnant women and immunocompromised persons
5. Avoid salicylates for 6 weeks postvaccination
6. Contraindicated in those with streptomycin allergy

Pneumococcal Vaccine

1. Local erythema and tenderness occur in 50% of patients
2. Systemic reactions are rare

Influenza Vaccine

1. Erythema and local tenderness common
2. Systemic reactions are rare (usually last 2 to 3 days)
3. Contraindicated in those with egg allergy
4. Does not increase risk of Guillain-Barre

Meningococcal Vaccine

1. Local reactions lasting 1 to 2 days
2. Systemic reactions (headache, malaise fatigue)
3. Fever $\geq$ 100°F [37.8°C (very small percentage of occurrences)]
4. Severe allergic reactions to a component of the vaccine or following a second dose is possible
5. Moderate or severe acute illness

Human Papillomavirus Vaccine

1. Mostly injection site tenderness and mild pain
2. No major systemic reactions yet reported

Reportable Events Following Vaccination

The Vaccine Adverse Events Reporting System (VAERS)

For all vaccines (including hepatitis A, hepatitis B, varicella, pneumococcal, and influenza):

1.	Monitor for any acute complications or sequelae of events including anaphylaxis, encephalopathy, or other life threatening conditions

Tetanus (in any combination)

1.	Anaphylaxis/anaphylactic shock: 7 days
2.	Brachial neuritis: 28 days

Pertussis (in any combination)

1.	Anaphylaxis/anaphylactic shock: 7 days
2.	Encephalopathy/encephalitis: 7 days

MMR (in any combination)

1.	Anaphylaxis: 7 days
2.	Encephalopathy/encephalitis: 7 days

Rubella (in any combination)

1.	Chronic arthritis: 42 days

Measles (in any combination)

1.	Thrombocytopenic purpura: 7 to 30 days
2.	Vaccine strain measles viral infection in immunodeficient recipient: 6 months

OPV

1.	Paralytic polio and Vaccine-strain polio viral infection:
	a.	Non-immunodeficient: 30 days
	b.	Immunodeficient: 6 months
	c.	Vaccine associated community case: No limit

IPV

1.	Anaphylaxis: 7 days

Hepatitis B

1.	Anaphylaxis: 7 days

Rotavirus

1.	Intussusception: 30 days

Sample Questions

1. The influenza vaccine is recommended for which age group?

    a. All children, regardless of age
    b. Annually, for children beginning at 6 months of age
    c. It is actually contraindicated for children with seasonal allergies.
    d. 2, 4, and 6 months of age

2. Which of the following is true about DtaP?

    a. Children should get 4 doses of DTaP, one dose at each of the following ages: 2, 4, 6, and 4 to 6 years.
    b. Children should get 5 doses of DTaP, one dose at each of the following ages: 2, 4, 6, 4 to 6 years, and age 12.
    c. Children should get 5 doses of DTaP, one dose at each of the following ages: 2, 4, 6, and 15 to 18 months and 4 to 6 years.
    d. Children should get 3 doses of DTaP, one dose at each of the following ages: 2, 4, 6, 4 to 6 years.

3. Children younger than 6 weeks of age should not get the Hib conjugate (Hib) vaccine because:

    a. A dose given at this time may reduce the infant's response to subsequent doses.
    b. A dose given at this time will not offer protection due to the influence of mother's hormones.
    c. A dose given at this time can actually cause serious sides effects.
    d. Before age 6 weeks, there is not enough adipose tissue for this vaccine.

Answers

1. Correct Answer: B

The flu vaccine is recommended for children beginning at 6 months of age. Allergies to eggs are contraindicated.

2. Correct Answer: C

There are 4 combination vaccines used to prevent diphtheria, tetanus and pertussis: DTaP, Tdap, DT, and Td. Two of these (DTaP and DT) are given to children younger than 7 years of age, and 2 (Tdap and Td) are given to older children and adults. Several other combination vaccines contain DTaP along with other childhood vaccines. Children should get 5 doses of DTaP, 1 dose at each of the following ages: 2, 4, 6, and 15 to 18 months and 4 to 6 years. DT does not contain pertussis and is used as a substitute for DTaP for children who cannot tolerate the pertussis vaccine. Td is a tetanus-diphtheria vaccine given to adolescents as a booster shot every 10 years, or after an exposure to tetanus under some circumstances. Tdap is similar to Td but also contains protection against pertussis. A single dose of Tdap is recommended for adolescents 11 or 12 years of age, or in place of one Td booster in older adolescents.

3. Correct Answer: A

Children younger than 6 weeks of age should not get the Hib vaccine because a dose given at this time may reduce the infant's response to subsequent doses.

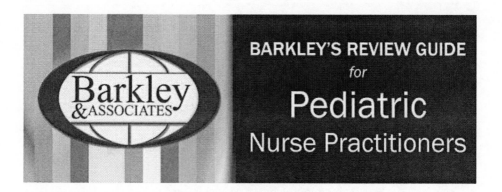

BARKLEY'S REVIEW GUIDE

for

Pediatric

Nurse Practitioners

Genetic Evaluations

Genetic Advancements

Genetic disorders are rare.

1. Major malformations occur in approximately 2% of live births
   a. Of these, 80% are associated with a genetic cause and an increased risk of recurrence
2. Only 40 to 45% of genetic disorders are diagnosed in the neonatal period
3. About 80% are identified before the age of six months

Indications for Genetic Evaluation

1. Advanced parental age (female and male)
2. History of miscarriages or stillbirths
3. Family history of:
   a. Birth defects
   b. Mental retardation
   c. Growth retardation
   d. Neurologic conditions
   e. Familial condition
4. Fetal exposure to:
   a. Medications
   b. Intrauterine infections
   c. Radiation
   d. Toxic chemicals
   e. Illegal substances
5. Ethnic background can increase the risk of carrier status for specific genetic disorders [e.g., sickle cell disease, phenylketonuria (PKU), etc.]
6. Phenotypic Presentation specific to genetic disorder, may include:
   a. Dysmorphic features
   b. Developmental delay
   c. Normal intelligence to mental retardation
   d. Short stature
   e. Failure to thrive
   f. Progressive deterioration of health status

  g.   Seizures

Genetic Assessment

1.   Obtain a pedigree history: Three generations
      a.   Family members: Including miscarriages and stillbirths
            i.   Gestational age
            ii.   Abnormalities
      b.   Health and mental status of each member
            i.   Specific information associated with disorder in question
            ii.   Current age
2.   Prenatal Screening and Diagnosis
      a.   Chorionic villus sampling (CVS): Eight to 12 weeks gestation (to
            detect chromosomal, biochemical, and DNA abnormalities)
      b.   Amniocentesis: Early 11 to 14 weeks; for second trimester
            diagnosis: 15 to 18 weeks (to detect chromosomal, biochemical,
            and DNA abnormalities)
      c.   Ultrasound: Throughout pregnancy (fetal structures best viewed
            after 12 weeks)
      d.   α-fetoprotein (AFP): After 14 weeks gestation
            i.   If elevated: Risk for fetal neural tube or body wall defects
            ii.   If low: Associated with increased risk of Down syndrome
                  1.   Maternal serum screening (MSAFP)
                  2.   Amniotic fluid α-fetoprotein (AFAFP)
      e.   Triple/Quad screening: After 14 weeks gestation (varied levels of
            each factor may indicate risk of Down syndrome, trisomy 18, or
            other chromosome abnormalities)
            i.   AFP
            ii.   β human chorionic gonadotropin (HGC)
            iii. Estriol
            iv.   Inhibin-A: Protein produced by the placenta and ovaries,
                  increased indicates a greater likehood of Down
                  syndrome; sensitivity to the detection of Down syndrome
                  is made stronger by the addition of Inhibin-A
      f.   Acetylcholinesterase: After 14 weeks gestation (if elevated, risk
            for neural tube defects)
      g.   Fetoscopy: Second trimester (to detect chromosomal,
            biochemical and DNA abnormalities from fetal blood; subtle
            abnormalities associated with disorders from fetal structures)
      h.   Precutaneous umbilical blood sampling (PUBS): Second trimester
            (to detect chromosomal, biochemical, and DNA abnormalities)

Genetic Disorders

Genetic Factors

A variety of chromosomal abnormalities, collectively known as "syndromes," may develop as a result of either parent's genetic influence. All other domains and factors being optimal, the influence of a genetic abnormality may significantly alter typical growth and development.

Trisomy 21 (Down Syndrome)

2. Presence of a third #21 chromosome
3. Occurs in 1:660 births
4. Increased maternal age increases risk
5. Degree of retardation may range from mild to severe
6. Typical physical findings
   a. Microcephaly, abnormal head shape
   b. Flattened nose: Frequently Down syndrome infants appear to have eyes set wider apart than usual. The appearance of hypertelorism is due to their flattened nose.
   e. **Hypertelorism (widely separated eyes)**
   f. **Hypotelorism (narrowly separated eyes)**
   c. Protruding tongue
   d. Inner epicanthal folds
   e. Upward slanting eyes
   f. Short broad hands/fingers; single palmar crease
   g. Delayed growth/development
   h. Hypotonia
7. Other manifestations that may occur
   a. Seizures
   b. Congenital heart disease
   c. Endocrine abnormalities
   d. Esophageal/duodenal atresia
   e. Hearing/vision impairment
   f. Obesity

Fragile X syndrome (Martin-Bell syndrome; Marker X syndrome)

1. Due to a change in the long arm of the X chromosome
2. Occurs in 1:2,000 males/1:4,000 females
3. 25% males asymptomatic carriers
4. Most common form of inherited mental retardation
5. Typical findings
   a. Large forehead/prominent jaw
   b. Macro-orchidism
   c. Avoidance of eye contact
   d. Developmental delay

     e.   Poor motor coordination
     f.   Hyperactivity
     g.   Seizures in up to 50% of patients

47 XXY syndrome (Klinefelter's syndrome)

1. A syndrome involving only males
2. Extra X chromosome
3. Appears normal at birth
4. Occurs in 1:1,000 males
5. Becomes apparent in puberty; may present initially as infertility
6. Most common cause of hypogonadism and infertility in men
7. Not inherited
8. Typical manifestations
     a.   Tall stature
     b.   Simian crease
     c.   Abnormal body proportions
     d.   Underdeveloped secondary sexual characteristics
     e.   Gynecomastia
     f.   Learning disability
     g.   Personality impairment

Trisomy 18 (Edward's syndrome)

1. Occurs in 1:3,000 births
2. Affect girls more often than boys
3. Majority of infants die before age 1 year
4. May be diagnosed in utero
5. Typical manifestations
     a.   History of pregnant uterus appearing unusually large
     b.   Low birth weight
     c.   Microcephaly
     d.   Low set ears
     e.   Micrognathia
     f.   Cryptorchidism
     g.   Hernias
     h.   Congenital heart disease
     i.   Kidney abnormalities
     j.   Ophthalmic manifestations
     k.   Mental retardation

XO Karyotype (Turner's syndrome)

1. Occurs in 1:2,000 live births
2. Most common sex-chromosome anomaly of females
3. Many embryos do not survive to term
4. Typical findings
     a.   Lymphadema

  b. Webbed neck
  c. Low hairline
  d. Learning disabilities
  e. Lack of secondary sexual characteristics
  f. "Shield" shaped chest (Wide-spaced)
  g. Variety of head/neck abnormalities
  h. Hypertension

Prader-Willi Syndrome

1. Occurs in 1:25,000
2. Generally sporadic occurrence
3. Empiric recurrence risk 1.6% (if already have a Prader-Willi syndrome child)
4. Typical findings
5. Hypotonia
  a. Poor sucking ability
  b. Almond-shaped palpebral fissures
  c. Small stature
  d. Insatiable appetite
  e. Behavioral problems beginning in childhood
  f. Below normal intelligence to mental retardation

Hemophilia A (X-Linked Recessive)

1. Occurs in 1:7,000 males
2. Deficiency of factor VIII
3. Female carriers (Mendelian distribution) have a:
  a. 25% risk of having an affected son with each pregnancy
  b. 25% risk of having a carrier daughter
  c. 25% chance of having a non-carrier daughter or healthy son
4. Frequency of carrier females is about 1:3,500
5. Severe form occurs in about 48% of cases
6. Typical findings
  a. Phenotypically normal at birth
  b. Bleeding tendency: Ranges from spontaneous bleeding to bleeding after trauma

Other Syndromes of Note

Marfan's syndrome

1. Inherited connective tissue disorder affecting skeletal, cardiac, and ophthalmic body systems
2. Occurs in 1:20,000 births
3. Tall statute
4. Arm span exceeds height
5. Thin extremities and fingers

6. Long narrow face
7. Pectus carinatum or excavatum
8. Hyperextension of joints
9. Genu recurvatum
10. Kyphoscoliosis
11. High arched, narrow palate
12. Aortic regurgitation
13. Mitral valve prolapse
14. Ectopia lentis
15. Iridodonesis

Tay-Sachs disease

1. Found in the Ashkenazic Jewish population
2. Occurs in 1:2,500 live births
3. Normal at birth; deterioration begins at ages three to six months
4. Typical findings
   a. Decreased muscle tone
   b. Listlessness
   c. Blindness
   d. Deafness
   e. Seizures
   f. Dementia
   g. Vegetative state
   h. Death
5. Can occur later as juvenile or adult onset forms, but this is rare

DiGeorge Syndrome/Anomaly

1. Congenital immunodeficiency characterized by abnormal facies, congenital heart defects, hypoparathyroidism with hypocalcemia, cognitive/behavioral psychiatric problems, and susceptibility to infection; a genetic condition characterized by abnormal pharyngeal arch development that results in defective development of the parathyroid glands, thymus, and the conotruncal region of the heart
2. Significant neonatal morbidity and mortality associated with cardiac defects
3. Typical findings
   a. Cellular immunity deficit leading to severe infections (thymus aplasia)
   b. Severe hypocalcemia and seizures in infancy (hypoparathyroidism)
   c. Aortic arch anomalies (conotruncal cardiac anomaly)
   d. Lateral displacement of inner canthi
   e. Short palpebral fissures
   f. Short philtrum

g.   Micrognathia
h.   Ear anomalies

Sample Questions

1. All of the following pose a potential for genetic problems except:

    a. Advanced parental age
    b. Family history of birth defects
    c. Previous premature pregnancies
    d. Fetal exposure to intrauterine infections

2. A 10-year-old girl presents with a history of short stature. Upon physical exam, the practitioner also finds a high arched palate, lymphedema of the hands, a low hairline, and a webbed neck. The parents also report some learning difficulties at school. These findings lead the practitioner to suspect which genetic condition?

    a. Growth hormone deficiency
    b. Turner syndrome
    c. Edwards syndrome
    d. Developmental delay

3. Infants with Down syndrome have a specific appearance at birth, such as inner epicanthal folds, hypotonia, and a protruding tongue. Other manifestations that may occur include all of the following except:

    a. Congenital heart defects
    b. Failure to thrive
    c. Seizures
    d. Hearing or vision impairment

Answers

1. Correct Answer: C
Advanced parental age, family history of birth defects, and fetal exposure to intrauterine infections all increase the risk of genetic problems. Previous premature pregnancies are not a genetic risk problem.

2. Correct Answer: B
These are all clinical manifestations of Turner syndrome. Approximately 1/3 of females are diagnosed in mid-childhood in the course of evaluation for short stature.

3. Correct Answer: B
Congenital heart defects, seizures, and hearing or vision impairments may occur with Down syndrome. Obesity, not failure to thrive, is also a manifestation.

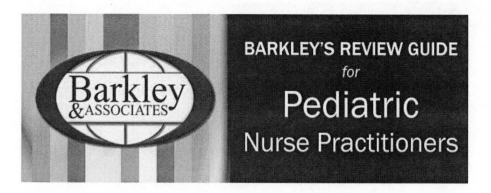
Disaster Planning Considerations

1.   Children cannot be treated as small adults
2.   Children have many unique anatomic, physiologic, immunologic, developmental, and psychological differences (please note the younger the infant or child, the more distinct the various system differences are from the older child and adult)
3.   Children experience increased vulnerability and response to disaster

Anatomic Differences

Size

Children are more vulnerable to exposure and toxicity (i.e. agents that are heavier or closer to ground than air such as sarin gas and chlorine).

Small Body Mass

1.   Less fat, less elastic connective tissue, and close proximity of the chest to abdominal organs
2.   Flying objects, falls, blunt or blast trauma may result in increased injury to multiple organs
        a.   Body surface area (BSA) to mass ratio is highest at birth and diminishes with age
        b.   BSA area of head to the limbs is higher, affecting burn injuries and hypothermia management
        c.   The higher BSA leads to more rapid absorption and systemic effects of toxins absorbed through thinner, less keratinized, highly permeable skin

Smaller Circulating Blood Volume/Less Fluid Reserve

1.   Even small amounts of volume loss may lead to hemorrhagic shock in the child
2.   Children are more vulnerable to bacterial agents; Staphylococcal enterotoxins and *Vibrio cholerae* lead to diarrhea/vomiting, hypovolemic

dehydration, and shock, especially in infants, small children, and children with special health care needs

Skeletal

1. Bones are more pliable, incompletely calcified skeletal system with active growth centers more susceptible to fracture
2. Orthopedic injuries often are missed in preverbal children (less than 7 years)
3. Additional organ damage (e.g., cardiac, lung) without incurred rib fractures are common and may be present
4. Cervical spine distortions may render x-ray interpretation as confusing; spinal cord injury may be noted without x-ray abnormalities

Head

1. Larger and heavier head compared to body proportion, accounting for a larger BSA than in the adult
2. A major heat loss source
3. Short neck and lacking well-developed musculature are common
4. The cranium is thinner and vulnerable to penetrating injury
5. The brain, which doubles in size by 6 months and is 80% of adult size by age 2, continues to do the following, which are risks for arrest and permanent changes:
    a. Mylenization
    b. Synapse formation
    c. Neuronal plasticity
    d. Biochemical stability

Chest

1. Mobile, pliable and offers little protection
    a. Risk of compromising cardiovascular flow, significant blood loss, and hypovolemic shock

Airway

1. Tongue is relatively large to oropharynx, creating potential for obstruction
2. Airway is narrower and angular, leading to difficulties with intubation needs
3. Lungs are smaller and subject to barotraumas resulting in a pneumothorax

Physiological Differences

Circulatory System

1. Compensates with raising heart rate and respirations during the early phase of hypovolemic shock (false impression of normalcy leads toward too little fluid resuscitation)

      a.   May be followed by a precipitous deterioration with little warning

Temperature Stability and Regulation

1. Affected by BSA-to-mass ratio, thin skin, lack of subcutaneous tissues with evaporative heat loss, and increased caloric/energy expenditures
2. Hypothermia is a significant risk factor for poor outcomes
3. Use of thermal blankets, warmed resuscitation rooms and fluids, and warmed inhaled gases may be required

Ventilation

Effects

1. Infants and young children have a higher minute ventilation per kilogram of body weight than adults and thus, can be exposed to relatively larger doses of aerosolized biological and chemical agents
2. More likely to feel effects and absorb more of the toxins from the lungs prior to clearing with ventilation
3. Resuscitation with fluids, drugs, and equipment are based on weight
4. The use of the Broselow/Hinkle pediatric resuscitation measuring tape is recommended for quick assessment
5. Fluids need to be administered with caution due to large volumes of hypotonic fluid that may place the child at risk for hyponatremia and seizures

Glycogen (Energy) Stores

A limited store of glycogen with higher relative metabolism puts children at risk for hypoglycemia

Immunologic Differences

1. An immature immunologic system creates a greater risk of infection
2. Less herd immunity from infections such as smallpox, and a unique susceptibility to some agents such as Venezuelan equine encephalitis

Developmental Differences

1. Limited verbal abilities: May not be able to describe symptoms or localize pain
2. Dependent on caretakers; may be more vulnerable to food source limitations when they are unavailable or contaminated
3. Limited motor skills to escape injury
4. Limited cognitive abilities to figure out how to flee from danger, follow directions from others, or even recognize a threat
5. Emotionally unstable due to the developing brain, especially in stressful encounters

6.   Reactions to danger and threats may be dictated by developmental stage
7.   There are additional concerns when the child has special health care needs that require interventions

Psychological Differences:

1.   Often gain cues from the caretakers or adults available to them; parental fears and feelings may impact and magnify their emotions
2.   Developmental stage alters emotions:

    a.   Younger children may exhibit regressive behaviors, increased temper tantrums, symptoms of clinginess, and difficulty with separation or sleep, which may increase crying, irritability, separation anxiety, and hyperactive startle responses

    b.   School-age children may exhibit depression, anger, and despair, which may be exacerbated by unrealistic fears of parents, families, and friends; school problems, physical somatizations (e.g., headache and stomach ache) may occur

    c.   Adolescents (due to the dramatic and complex physical, psychological, and social transition) may be vulnerable to the development of major psychiatric disorders such as depression; also, risk taking behavior (e.g., alcohol, tobacco and other drug usage or suicide) may surface, as adolescents often hide their feelings or symptoms for fear of being perceived as abnormal

Sample Questions

1. You are responsible for the planning and implementation of a disaster preparedness education program and policy at your clinic. Which of the following is the most important factor to keep in mind when formulating and educating people regarding the policy?

   a. Expect toddlers and preschoolers to display regressive behaviors, more temper tantrums, and experience difficulty with separation in the event of a disaster

   b. Show school age children visual images and explain in detail what to expect

   c. Assess adolescents for abnormal behaviors during this time such as fear, anxiety, and force them to express their feelings

   d. Parents should not hide their emotions, fear, and anxiety about the event with their children

2. A 10-month-old is asleep upstairs when an unexpected natural disaster strikes the home. The family evacuation plan requires that all family members remain in the center of the home away from any windows until they no longer feel they are in eminent danger. The 10-month-old is most vulnerable during this time because of developmental differences in which of the following categories?

   a. Motor
   b. Cognitive
   c. Language
   d. Moral

3. In assessing cardiac output and circulation in a pediatric emergency, the provider should:

   a. Listen for an apical pulse rather than palpate
   b. Rely on capillary refill time for children both warm or cold
   c. Take the peripheral pulse as a reliable assessment of perfusion
   d. Use the color of the extremities to assess perfusion

Answers

1. Correct Answer: A

In choice A, toddlers will regress and exhibit changes as described; this is an expected finding and should not be a cause for alarm. Parents can provide support to children and assist them in getting through this difficult time. In choice B, children (even those in school) should not be shown visual images that may scare or cause increased anxiety. In addition, a parent should provide an avenue for open communication and answer all questions but avoid bombarding and overwhelming the child with every detail of the event. In choice C, it is expected that adolescents will exhibit fear and anxiety during this time of change. Parents should be supportive and encourage, but not force, expression of feelings. In choice D, while parents should not hide things from their children, it is important to realize that a parent's fears or anxiety can impact and magnify the emotions of a child.

2. Correct Answer: A

Although the child has limitations in cognitive and language development, at this time, it is the limited motor abilities that prevent her from escaping injury. Moral development does not yet apply and is not as applicable to this situation.

3. Correct Answer: C

Because capillary refill time can be misleading in a child who is cold, a peripheral pulse is considered a more reliable assessment of perfusion. Those patients who have palpable peripheral pulses are then assessed for their mental status.

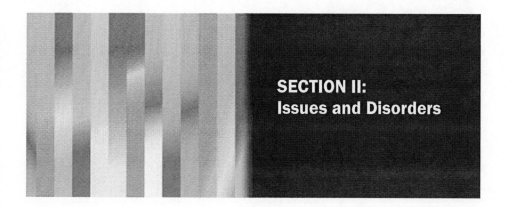

SECTION II:
Issues and Disorders

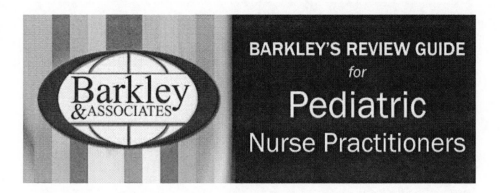

BARKLEY'S REVIEW GUIDE
for
Pediatric
Nurse Practitioners

Infant Health Issues and Disorders

Disorders That May Be Present at Birth

Rubella

Cardiovascular, ophthalmic complications

Cytomegalovirus (CMV)

Microcephaly, sensorineural hearing loss, chorioretinitis

Herpes

Skin, mouth, ophthalmic, central nervous systems (CNS), pulmonary manifestations

Congenital syphilis

Hepatitis, hemolytic anemia, nephrosis, myocarditis, bony findings, cystic fibrosis

Sudden Infant Death Syndrome (SIDS)

The sudden, unexplained death of an infant under 1 year of age

1.   Death remains unexplained despite a thorough investigation of all circumstances

Causes/Incidence
1.   Cause unknown
2.   Occurs in 5,000 babies annually
3.   Peak incidence age is 2 to 4 months

Signs/Symptoms
1.   Infant is found unexpectedly dead
2.   Unresponsive to resuscitative efforts
3.   No clues are evident to suggest SIDS
4.   Occurs in previously healthy infants

Differential Diagnosis

1. Intracranial hemorrhage
2. Abuse
3. Accident
4. Suffocation
5. Myocarditis

Diagnostic Studies

1. None

Management

1. Reduce risk
   a. Baby should sleep on its back
   b. Avoid soft bedding, waterbeds, deep blankets, and over-bundling
   c. Avoid passive smoking
   d. Breastfeed
   e. Keep room comfortable but not too warm
   f. Apnea monitor for high risk infants
2. Emotional support

Failure to Thrive (FTT)

Typically used to represent an infant whose weight falls > 2 percentiles below or whose absolute length/weight are below the 5th percentile

1. No global definition exists
2. May be organic or non-organic

Causes/Incidence

1. Predisposing medical conditions
2. Poverty
3. Neglect
4. Mental illness
5. Affects males and females equally

Signs/Symptoms

1. Weight as described in definition
2. Decreased intake
3. Increased losses
4. Increased needs
5. Other symptoms of medical disorder
6. Avoidance of human interaction in non-organic causes
   a. Seeks human contact
   b. Odd affect: No expression
   c. Avoids eye contact

Differential Diagnoses

1.   Organic (medical) causes
      a.   Gastrointestinal (GI) disease/disorders
      b.   Cardiopulmonary disease
      c.   Hormonal insufficiency
      d.   Infectious disease
      e.   Mental retardation
      f.   Lead poisoning
2.   Non-organic (human interaction) causes
      a.   Purposeful abuse/neglect
      b.   Poverty
      c.   Parents' knowledge and/or skills deficit

Diagnostic Studies

1.   As indicated to rule out underlying disease
2.   At least 2 weight measures required
3.   Home evaluation

Management

1.   Dependent upon cause

Fever of the Very Young Infant

Defined as a rectal temperature of 100.4°F (38°C)

1.   The most common manifestation of infection
2.   In the very young infant, temperatures can be subnormal with infection
3.   Elevations of 104°F (40°C) are commonly found with minor infections such as minor respiratory infections, otitis media, or infectious diarrhea
4.   Temperatures over 104°F (40°C) are more commonly associated with severe illnesses such as pneumonia or meningitis
5.   Other causes of fever in the very young infant include the inability to thermoregulate, as well as others

Common Misconceptions about Fever

Misconception	Prolonged high fever in infants can cause brain damage
	There is no medical evidence that this is true; brain damage results if body temperature rises above 107°F (41.7°C); the body mechanisms will not allow the temperature from fever to rise above 106°F (41.1°C)
Misconception	Any temperature above core body temperature may be a fever
	This is not so in children
Misconception	A high temperature can cause convulsions
	Febrile convulsions can occur at temperature elevations as low as 101°F (38.3°C); such is a phenomenon of how quickly the temperature rises, not how high it goes
Misconception	Teething and its relationship to causing fever in children is controversial
	Usually fever in a teething child is a sign of an underlying infection

Fever in Early Infancy (the first 2 months of life)

1. Temperatures higher than 101.8°F (38.9°C) suggest a serious bacterial infection (36% of patients); fever in the first 2 months of life is uncommon but if present, it is frequently serious
2. 40% of fevers occur in infants less than 4 weeks of age
3. In 40% of cases, the cause is viral
    a. The most common are enteroviruses and herpes simplex
    b. Enteroviruses have a peak in activity between July and September
4. Bacterial infections, common organisms
    a. First month: Group B streptococcus (GBS) and gram-negative enteric organisms
    b. Second month: S. pneumoniae and H. influenzae
    c. Note: Serious infections can result in bacteremia, which is more than twice as frequent in the first month (7.4%) as in the second month (3.1%)

Assess the Degree of Illness

1. Mildly ill infants appear alert and active, smile, and feed well
2. Moderately ill infants may be fussy or irritable but continue to feed, are consolable and may smile; these infants may have otitis media

3.   Severely ill infants [temperatures of 104°F (40°C) or higher] appear listless, cannot be consoled, feed poorly or not at all; severely ill infants may also have vomiting with abdominal distention, a history of apnea, seizures, or exhibit signs of shock
     a.   These infants should be admitted to the hospital
     b.   Infants less than 4 weeks of age and older high risk infants (e.g., those with underlying cardiac or pulmonary disease or a history of a prolonged or complicated nursery stay) should also be admitted

4.   Negative lab screenings are still recommended in some centers and includes:
     a.   White blood cell count of 5,000 to 15,000
     b.   A band count less than 1,500

5.   When a local site of infection cannot be found, consider the diagnosis of urinary tract infection (UTI)
     a.   Found in 3% of febrile infants
     b.   10% of patients with UTI have bacteremia

6.   Risk for meningitis with fever
     a.   Enteroviral meningitis occurs in 10% to 39% of febrile infants
     b.   Frequency of bacterial meningitis is 1% to 2%
     c.   Causative agents include: Group *B streptococcus, S. pneumoniae, H. influenzae, Salmonella, N. Meningitis*, and *E. coli*

7.   Occult bacteremia
     a.   Incidence of occult bacteremia varies with age and the height of temperature
     b.   Major causative pathogens:
          i.   *Streptococcus pneumoniae* (40 to 73%)
          ii.   *Haemophilus influenzae* type B (11 to 40%)
          iii.   *Neisseria meningitidis* (less than 1 to 5%)
     c.   Toxic-appearing infants less than 12 weeks have a higher probability of having a serious bacterial infection
          i.   Toxic is defined as a clinical presentation congruent with the sepsis syndrome (e.g., lethargy, signs of poor perfusion, or marked hypoventilation, hyperventilation or cyanosis)
          ii.   Lethargy is defined as a level of consciousness characterized by poor or absent eye contact, the failure of the child to recognize parents, or the failure to interact with persons or objects in the environment

Low-Risk Criteria for Serious Infection

1.   Previously healthy
2.   Nontoxic appearance
3.   No clinical evidence of a focal bacterial infection
4.   Negative lab screening

Management

1.   Most commonly used drugs
     a.   Ibuprofen (approved after 6 months of age)
     b.   Acetaminophen
2.   Clinical trials of both drugs
     a.   Equal efficacy of both medications at:
          i.   Ibuprofen dosed at 10 mg/kg
          ii. Acetaminophen dosed at 15 mg/kg
               Note: The movement away from the use of aspirin over
               the past 20 years has been due to the association of
               aspirin and developing Reye's syndrome
3.   Treating fever should be done on a case-by-case basis; some experts
     believe that reduction in fever impairs antibody production, which in turn,
     delays recovery from infection
4.   First-line treatment for fever is acetaminophen
     a.   Because the main effect of acetaminophen is in CNS, it does not
          have the same side effects associated with aspirin and other
          nonsteroidal anti-inflammatory drugs (NSAIDs)
     b.   10 to 15 mg/kg every 4 to 6 hours
     c.   Maximum per day dose: 50 to 75 mg/kg
     d.   Doses > 140 mg/kg can be toxic if used for several days
5.   Combination use of ibuprofen and acetaminophen
     a.   No studies show superior effects when both are used
     b.   Risk for toxicity remains unknown
     c.   Studies show increased risk for error in dosing
          i.   Some studies suggest more than half of the participants
               were given incorrect amounts of antipyretics; infants < 1
               year old were more likely to receive an inaccurate dose;
               however, parents who stated that the medication dosage
               was based on weight were more likely to give the correct
               amount of the medication
          ii. Errors also occur because parents can become confused
               about the timing to give ibuprofen and acetaminophen

Sample Questions

1. The main causes of death in infants less than 1 year of age include which of the following?

    a. Suffocation, child abuse, drowning, and burns
    b. Suffocation, motor vehicle crashes, drowning, and burns
    c. Suffocation, motor vehicle crashes, drowning, and poisoning
    d. Suffocation, motor vehicle crashes, falling from chairs and other high places, and burns

2. You are examining a 2-month-old and hear a heart murmur. You explain to the child's mother that the murmur is most likely harmless and do not make a referral to a cardiologist. What would be your best rationale?

    a. The murmur is heard in diastole and is of no concern.
    b. The child appears healthy, and this is likely a patent ductus arteriosus that is closing.
    c. The murmur is loudest when the child is standing
    d. The murmur is systolic, Grade I or II, and has no thrill.

3. Which of the following statements is true about fever in the very young infant?

    a. Fevers must be over 101.8°F (38.9°C) to cause febrile seizures.
    b. Fever in the first couple of months of life is common.
    c. Fever of the very young infant is defined as a rectal temperature of 100.4 °F (38°C).
    d. Fever of temperatures 104°C (40°C) or higher can be meaningless in the infant.

Answers

1. Correct Answer: B

Suffocation, motor vehicle crashes, drowning and fires/burns are the leading causes of unintentional injury death among babies less than 1 year old.

2. Correct Answer: D

Innocent murmurs are always systolic, Grade I or II, and have no thrill. Innocent murmurs like a pulmonic ejection murmur, Still's murmur, or venous hum are always systolic, Grade I or II, loudest when recumbent or after exercise, and have no thrill.

3. Correct Answer: C

For fever in early infancy (first 2 months of life), temperatures higher than 101.8°F (38.9°C) suggest serious bacterial infection (36%). Fever in the first 2 months of life is uncommon but if present, it is frequently serious. Severely ill infants [temperature of 104°F (40°C) or higher] appear listless, cannot be consoled, and feed poorly or not at all. These infants should be admitted to the hospital. Febrile convulsions can occur at temperature elevations as low as 101°F (38.3°C). How quickly the temperature rises is an important consideration, but how high it goes is not necessarily.

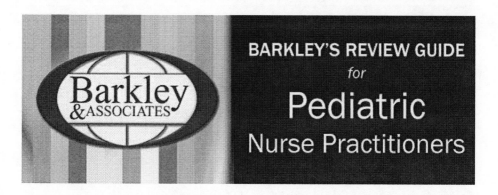

Toddler and Preschool Issues and Disorders

Stuttering

Abnormal speech patterns characterized by repetitions and pauses in speech

Causes/Incidence

1. Cause is debatable but generally believed to be developmental dysfluency
2. Occurs more often in males
3. Occurs in up to 10% of children at some point and over one-half recover spontaneously
4. There may be an increased incidence in families with a history of abnormal speech

Signs/Symptoms

1. Repetition of sounds
2. Pauses within or between words
3. Other speech and language problems may be present
4. Initial speech development without incidence as stuttering occurs later
5. Lasts for several weeks to 6 months but often resolves without intervention

Differential Diagnosis

1. Hearing impairment
2. Visual impairment

Diagnostic Studies

1. None: Clinical diagnosis

Management

1. Ignore initial presentation
2. Encourage parents to be patient
3. Refer if:
   a. Stuttering lasts > 6 months
   b. Child avoids speaking

Pervasive Development Disorder

A disorder characterized by altered response to environmental stimuli and impaired social interactions. The term encompasses a collection of disorders including autism, atypical autism, Rett's disorder, Asperger's syndrome, childhood disintegrative disorder, and conditions that are collectively known as autism spectrum disorders.

Distinguishing Features of Pervasive Developmental Disorders

According to the fourth edition of the Diagnostic and Statistic Manual of Mental Disorders (DSM-IV-TR):

1. Autistic disorder: Marked abnormal or impaired development in social interaction; there is also a greatly restrictive repertoire of activity and interests, usually noted within the first year of life
2. Asperger's syndrome: Severe and sustained impairment in social interaction and the development of restricted, repetitive patterns of behavior, interests, and activities; non-clinically significant delays in language acquisition
3. Rett's disorder: A specific and highly distinctive pattern of developmental regression following a period of normal functioning through the first 5 months after birth; has been diagnosed only in females
4. Childhood disintegrative disorder (CDD): Marked regression in multiple areas of functioning following a period of at least 2 years of apparently normal development
5. Pervasive developmental disorder (PDD) is not otherwise specified; severe and pervasive impairment in the development of reciprocal social interaction, but the criteria are not met for a specific pervasive developmental disorder

Predisposing Factors

1. Social environment in which causative factors are thought to include:
    a. Parental rejection
    b. Child responses to deviant parental personality characteristics
    c. Family breakup
    d. Family stress
    e. Insufficient stimulation
    f. Faulty communication patterns
2. Biological factors:
    a. Genetics; sibling and twin studies have revealed strong evidence that genetic factors play a significant role
3. Neurological factors:
    a. Maternal rubella
    b. Untreated phenylketonuria
    c. Tuberous sclerosis

      d.   Anoxia during birth
      e.   Encephalitis
      f.   Infantile spasms
4.   Central nervous system (CNS) diseases, such as mental retardation, congenital syphilis, epilepsy, and congenital rubella

Causes/Incidence

1.   Neurological disorder due to brain insult in utero
2.   No clear etiology and may include infection
3.   Occurs in 2 to 5 per 10,000 population
4.   Overall more common in males (except Rett's disorder)
5.   More severe when occurs in females

Signs/Symptoms

1.   Normal growth and development until 2 to 3 years
2.   Onset of developmental delay before age 3 is part of diagnostic criteria
3.   DSM-IV-TR requires 6 total behaviors from 3 categories (motor, language, communication and social); in autism, the child typically has speech and language delays; however, some demonstrate seemingly advanced speech but may use speech abnormally and inappropriately [i.e., echolalia (mechanical and meaningless repetition of another person's words)]
4.   May also see cognitive delays and learning delays
5.   Emotional unresponsiveness (even in infancy with lack of eye contact, and facial expressiveness)
6.   Range of symptom presentation varies

Differential Diagnosis

1.   Mental retardation
2.   Psychosis
3.   Genetic syndromes
4.   Expressive language disorder or mixed receptive-expressive language disorder
5.   Stereotypic movement disorder
6.   Attention deficit hyperactivity disorder
7.   Sensory impairment
8.   Selective mutism

Differential diagnosis is defined by the following components:

1.   Determine intellectual level
2.   Determine level of language development
3.   Consider whether child's behavior is appropriate for
      a.   Chronological age
      b.   Mental age
      c.   Language age

4.   If not appropriate, consider differential diagnosis of a psychiatric disorder according to:
     a.   Pattern of social interaction
     b.   Pattern of language
     c.   Pattern of play
     d.   Other behavior
5.   Identify any relevant medical conditions
6.   Consider whether there are any relevant psychosocial factors

Diagnostic Studies

1.   Electroencephalography (EEG) if seizures or language delay are present
2.   As indicated to rule out other symptoms
3.   May use behavior checklist, such as:
     a.   Autism Diagnostic Observation Schedule
     b.   Vineland Adaptive Behavior Scale
     c.   Autism Behavior Checklist
     d.   Checklist for Autism in Toddlers (CHAT)
     e.   Modified Checklist for Autism in Toddlers (MCHAT)

Management

1.   Early screening and referral is of extreme importance
2.   Treatment is individualized
3.   Refer for community resources, family support

Other Pervasive Disorders

Rett's Disorder:

A neurodegenerative disease affecting only females

1.   The age of onset is about 1
2.   Etiology is unknown
3.   Clinical presentation
     a.   Ceases to gain developmental milestones
     b.   CNS irritability and withdrawal develop
     c.   Loss of skills already mastered
           i.   Speech
           ii.   Hand skills
     d.   Stereotypic hand movements
     e.   Delayed head growth
     f.   Seizures
     g.   Scoliosis
     h.   Hypertonicity

Management

1.   Goal is to preserve functional abilities

a. Physical therapy
b. Occupational therapy
c. Speech therapy
d. Seizure management
e. Support of family
f. Referral to social services, if necessary

Childhood Disintegrative Disorder

1. The classification or diagnosis given to children who do not fit the criteria for the other pervasive developmental disorders
2. More males are affected than females; however, females who are affected exhibit a more severe form of the disorder

Asperger's Disorder

1. Has similar features as autism but speech is not affected
2. More males are affected; however, females that are affected have a more severe form of the disorder
3. Language Deficitis: Evaluate for Autism
   a. No babbling, pointing, or other gesturing by 12 months
   b. No single words by 16 months
   c. No 2 word spontaneous phrases by 24 months
   d. Loss of language (any age)
   e. Loss of social skills (any age)

Sample Questions

1. There are a multitude of developmental problems that the nurse practitioner must be alert and recognize due to the importance of early intervention. The term "pervasive development disorders," also called PDDs, refers to a group of conditions that involve delays in the development of many basic skills, most notably:

   a. Ability to cooperate, are typically depressive with flat affect and delayed motor skills
   b. Ability to socialize with others, to have fine motor skills, and to use imagination
   c. Ability to socialize with others and generally have problems in all areas of functioning
   d. Ability to socialize with others, to communicate, and to use imagination

2. Children with Rett's disorder have the symptoms associated with a PDD and also suffer problems with physical development. They generally suffer the loss of many motor or movement skills, such as use of their hands, and develop poor coordination. The disease almost never:

   a. Affects males
   b. Allows child to live to adulthood
   c. Is treatable with cognitive therapy
   d. All are correct

3. In the preschooler who begins stuttering, the initial presentation is usually ignored for a period of time. However, the child should be referred to a specialist if he continues to avoid speaking or if the stuttering lasts for more than:

   a. 3 months
   b. 6 months
   c. 9 months
   d. 1 year

Answers

1. Correct Answer:

D

The term "pervasive development disorders," also called PDDs, refers to a group of conditions that involve delays in the development of many basic skills, most notably the ability to socialize with others, to communicate, and to use imagination. Children with these conditions often are confused in their thinking and generally have problems understanding the world around them.

2. Correct Answer:

A

Children with this very rare disorder have the symptoms associated with a PDD and also suffer problems with physical development. They generally suffer the loss of many motor or movement, skills – such as walking and use of their hands – and develop poor coordination. This condition has been linked to a defect on the X chromosome, so it almost always affects girls.

3. Correct Answer:

B

Stuttering is indicated by a repetition of sounds or pauses within or between words. Other speech and language problems may be present, though initial speech development proceeds without incidence as stuttering occurs later. Stuttering often lasts for several weeks to 6 months and resolves without intervention. If this is not the case, a referral to a specialist is necessary.

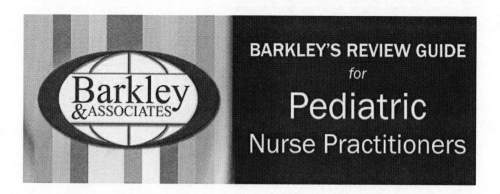

School Age and Adolescent Issues and Disorders

Obesity

A term generally used to describe a condition in which the body fat to lean mass ratio is too great as a result of high caloric intake and/or low energy use

1.   Obesity may be defined as mild, moderate or morbid

Causes/Incidence

1.   Usually a combination of physiologic, genetic, and environmental causes
2.   May be genetic predisposition
3.   Diet high in fats and simple carbohydrates
4.   Relative inactivity
5.   Use of food for emotional comfort or as a control mechanism
6.   Physical or genetic disorders of decreased energy expenditure
7.   As many as 30% of U.S. children are estimated to be obese

Signs/Symptoms

1.   Obesity as evidenced by one or more measures
2.   Parent or child concern
3.   Sad/depressed affect
4.   May be associated with a variety of mood manifestations

Differential Diagnosis

1.   Endocrine disease
2.   Prader-Willi syndrome
3.   Medication-induced obesity (antipsychotics)

Diagnostic Studies

1.   As indicated to rule out physical causes
2.   As indicated to assess for physiologic sequelae
3.   Determination of obesity:
      a.   Weight/height ratio 95th percentile
      b.   More than 120% of ideal body weight: Divide child's height and weight by 50th percentile height and weight and multiply by 100

    c.   Skin fold thickness above 85th percentile

    d.   Body mass index (BMI) is greater than 95th percentile for age/gender

Management

1. Prevention through anticipatory guidance
2. Treat underlying physical cause if appropriate
3. Goal for the younger child is to stabilize weight; linear growth will compensate
4. Nutritional planning
5. Increase activity
6. Counseling referral if psychosocial issues seem a likely cause

Child Abuse and Neglect

A collective term used to describe acts of commission and/or omission including physical, sexual and emotional acts that endanger the health and development of the child

1. All states have required reporting standards for suspected abuse/neglect by mandated professionals

Causes/Incidence

1. Abusers are usually former victims
2. Frequently there is psychiatric, cognitive or emotional impairment
3. Neglect is the most common form of child abuse
4. African Americans and Native Americans have twice the national average of reported incidence
5. 80% of abusers are parents
6. More than 1,000,000 cases are reported annually

Signs/Symptoms

1. History is vague and not compatible with the injury
2. Delay in seeking care can lead to fractures and bruises in various stages of healing
3. Soft tissue markings with outline of a hand, object, weapon, or cigarette burn
4. Physical needs not met
5. Developmental delays
6. Child/parent interaction is unusual

Differential Diagnosis

1. Accidents
2. Underlying disease
3. Homeopathic or cultural practices

Diagnostic Studies

1.   Thorough physical examination
2.   As indicated to rule out underlying causes of symptoms (e.g., coagulopathies and/or osteogenesis imperfecta)
3.   Home assessment
4.   Blood coagulation studies (platelet count, bleeding time, prothrombin time, and partial thromboplastin time) in children with bruises or a history of "easy bruising"
5.   Radiographic studies:
      a.   Local radiological evaluation in children with limited range of motion or bony tenderness on examination
      b.   Skeletal survey: For any child with soft tissue findings who is nonverbal or unable to give a clear history (more than 4 to 5 years of age) or for infants suspected of failure to thrive
      c.   CT scans/bone scans/MRI: On a case by case basis, depending on clinical findings
      d.   Ultrasonography is useful if visceral injury is suspected
6.   Serum calcium, phosphorus, and alkaline phosphatase levels may be useful if bone disease is suspected

Management

1.   Education and prevention
2.   Identify high risk mothers/parents and refer
3.   Anticipatory guidance
4.   Mandatory reporting according to state statute

Attention Deficit Hyperactivity Disorder (ADHD)

ADHD is the most commonly diagnosed behavioral problem in childhood and is now regarded as a chronic illness.

The essential impairment is a deficit behavioral inhibition which disrupts the developmental process of learning how to self-regulate behaviors. Instead, behaviors such as inattention, distractibility, impulsivity, and hyperactivity, which are appropriate behaviors in young children, persist into school-age and adolescence making internal regulation of behaviors difficult at best.

According to the fourth edition of the Diagnostic and Statistical Manual of Mental Disorders (DSM-IV), there are 3 diagnostic subtypes of ADHD:

1.   Predominantly inattentive type
2.   Predominantly hyperactive-impulsive type
3.   Combined type (most children are diagnosed with this type of ADHD)

Other essential elements must be present to make this diagnosis:

1. Symptoms must be present before the age of 7
2. Symptoms must persist for at least 6 months
3. Symptoms must be more frequent and more severe than those observed in other children at the same level of development
4. Symptoms interfere with functioning in at least two settings:
    a. Home
    b. School
    c. Play

Epidemiology

1. About 3 to 15% of school-aged children are affected
    a. 4% of primary care visits
    b. 50% in psychiatric visits
2. Boys are affected at a rate six times greater than girls
3. Wide variation in reported incidence due to diagnostic criteria and unique manifestations of symptoms by some children

Predisposing factors

1. Biological influences
    a. Genetics: Frequency among family members has been noted
    b. Biochemical theory: Implicates a deficit of dopamine and norepinephrine in the brain
    c. Areas of the brain affected include the frontal and prefrontal regions
    d. Prenatal factors include maternal smoking during pregnancy
    e. Perinatal factors include prematurity, signs of fetal distress, prolonged labor, and perinatal asphyxia
    f. Postnatal factors include cerebral palsy, epilepsy and central nervous system (CNS) trauma or infections
2. Environmental influences
    a. Environmental lead
    b. Dietary factors, including food dyes and additives and sugar
3. Psychosocial influences
    a. Disorganized or chaotic environments
    b. Child abuse or neglect
    c. Family history of alcoholism, hysterical, or sociopathic behaviors
    d. Developmental learning disorders

Causes/Incidence

1. Unknown
2. Not linked to foods, sugar or excess television
3. No longer believed to be a result of head injury or birth trauma
4. May be a linked to exposure to toxins in utero as a result of maternal drug, cigarette or alcohol use

Signs/Symptoms

1.   DSM IV-TR criteria require onset before age 7, lasting at least six months and causing a handicap in at least two settings of the life (e.g., home, school, etc.)
2.   Symptoms cannot be attributable to underlying psychiatric disease
3.   In addition to these, there must be at least 6 symptoms of inattention or 6 symptoms of hyperactivity/impulsivity

Clinical Manifestations of Core Symptoms

Inattention	Impulsivity	Hyperactivity
Make careless mistakes	Difficulties awaiting one's turn	Fidgetiness
Fails to pay attention to detail	Frequently blurts out answers	Difficulty remaining seated
Easily distracted	Interrupts or intrudes on others	Difficulty playing quietly
Difficulty concentrating long enough to complete task		Subjective feelings of restlessness in adolescents
Difficulties following instructions		Difficulties with social relationships
Difficulties organizing task and activities		Low frustration tolerance

Co-Morbidity

1.   Learning disabilities (35%)
2.   Psychiatric disorders
      a.   Anxiety (25%)
      b.   Depression (25%)
      c.   Oppositional defiant disorder or conduct disorder (50%)

Differential Diagnosis

1.   Sensory impairment
2.   Psychiatric disorder
3.   Age appropriate activity
4.   Situational anxiety

Diagnostic Studies

1.   Perinatal history

2.   A variety of standardized tests/questionnaires are used to assess symptoms
      a.   Connor's Rating Scales
      b.   ADHD rating scale
      c.   Achenbach Child Behavior Checklist
      d.   Vanderbilt Assessment Tool
3.   Direct observation in multiple settings

Management

Requires multi-modal management

1.   Structured environment
2.   Operant conditioning techniques
3.   Consider mental health referral
4.   Pharmacologic management:
      a.   CNS stimulants: Highly effective (70 to 90% effective)
            i.   Methylphenidates (e.g., Ritalin, Concerta, Metadate, Focalin)
            ii.   Amphetamines (e.g., Adderall, Adderrall XR, Dexadrine, Vyvanse)
            iii.   Stimulants increase availability of neurotransmitters to increase focus and attention
            iv.   Prescribing principles:
                  1.   Start low and go slow; titrate up at intervals of one week; get feedback from parents and teachers to assess effectiveness
                  2.   Behavior changes can be identified within 30 and 90 minutes of ingestion
                  3.   Short-acting preparations generally last four hours, and often need re-dosing; long-acting preparations generally last 10 to 12 hours
                  4.   Avoid evening dosage changes to minimize insomnia
5.   If a child does not respond to higher doses of one stimulant, or if side effects are unacceptable, switch to another stimulant before considering other medications
6.   Contraindications:
      a.   Symptomatic cardiovascular disease
      b.   Moderate hypertension
      c.   Marked anxiety
      d.   Glaucoma
      e.   History of drug abuse
      f.   Depression
      g.   Depression/suicide risk

7.   American Academy of Pediatrics (2006) recommends a baseline EKG prior to initiation of stimulants

8.   Long-acting stimulants cannot be chewed as it destroys the delivery system

9.   Ritalin
   a.   Most commonly used, usually prescribed first because it has the least side effects
   b.   Usual dose 0.3 to 0.7 mg/kg, starting with 5 to 10 mg in the morning
   c.   If not effective, increase dose in increments of 2.5 to 5.0 mg per week until effect level is reached
   d.   Once the effective dose is reached, it can be given in two or three doses per day
   e.   Weekend dosing is optional
   f.   If using a sustained-release form of medication, dosing is simplified

10.   Side Effects
   a.   Insomnia
   b.   Anorexia
   c.   Weight loss
   d.   Tachycardia
   e.   Temporary decrease in rate of growth and development
   f.   Tolerance to medication
   g.   Tics
   h.   Headaches
   i.   Stomach aches

11.   Second-line medications: Used especially with co-morbidities; unresponsive to stimulants
   i.   Selective norepinephrine inhibitor/SNRI [e.g., atomoxetine (Strattera)]
   ii.   Tricyclic antidepressants
   iii.   Alpha adrenergic agonists [(e.g., clonidine (Catapres), guanfacine (Tenex)]
   iv.   Selective serotonin reuptake inhibitors (SSRIs)

12.   Non-pharmacological management
   a.   May benefit from cognitive, social skills or parenting therapy
   b.   A "drug holiday" should be attempted periodically under direction of the prescriber to determine effectiveness of the medication and need for continuation

Eating Disorders

Chronic disturbances in eating patterns accompanied by distorted body image

1. Anorexia nervosa is characterized by eating disturbances, weight loss, and refusal to maintain body weight at 85% of expected weight for height; amenorrhea ensues
2. Bulimia nervosa is characterized by episodic binge and purge episodes
3. Cause is not clearly defined but is believed to arise from familial issues, social pressure low self-esteem, and a desire for control
4. Peak incidences are at age 14 and 18 years
5. Overall, mortality is as high as 10% as a combination of suicide and consequential death

Signs/Symptoms

1. Weight loss
2. Anemia
3. Amenorrhea
4. Dry skin
5. Constipation
6. Low vital signs
7. Lanugo
8. Evidence of self-induced vomiting

Differential Diagnosis

1. Organic disease producing weight loss
2. Pregnancy
3. Depression
4. Substance abuse

Laboratory/Diagnostics

1. As indicated to rule out organic disease
2. Mild malnutrition: < 20% below ideal body weight (IBW)
3. Moderate malnutrition: < 20 to 30% below IBW
4. Severe malnutrition: < 30% below IBW

Management

1. Interdisciplinary management
2. Behavior modification
3. Psychotherapy
4. May need hospitalization

Sample Questions

1. You are interviewing an 11-year-old child who says that her uncle has touched her "in places she doesn't like." You should proceed with care because oftentimes children:

   a. Do not want to "tattle"
   b. Frequently make things up for attention
   c. Feel they are at least in part responsible for sexual abuse
   d. Are not yet concrete thinkers, especially with regard to sexual matters

2. A 14-year-old girl comes in for her annual check-up accompanied by her mother. Upon first seeing the girl, you observe that she has stained teeth, callused knuckles, and that she is hoarse. You will want to work Jennifer up for:

   a. Personality disorder
   b. Substance abuse
   c. Bulimia nervosa
   d. Anorexia nervosa

3. It is often difficult for to diagnose attention deficit hyperactivity disorder (ADHD), as it may look like another condition. The differential for ADHD would include:

   a. Substance abuse, anxiety, conduct disorder
   b. Depression, bipolar disorder, Tourette syndrome
   c. Anxiety, conduct disorder, mental retardation
   d. All of the above

Answers

1. Correct Answer: C

Although still primarily concrete thinkers, as children advance through the latency age years, they become better able to understand concepts and symbolism. They still tend to want their emotional support to be family oriented, but socialization is with their peers, usually of the same sex. By the early school years, children are able to orient themselves in time and space, especially relating to events and holidays, and draw simplistic floor plans of the place where the abuse occurred. They are capable of deceiving in a more convincing way and are more capable of keeping a secret. As they become more aware of the unacceptable nature of sexual touching, and since they are too young to control their environment well, many children of this age feel they are responsible at least in part for the sexual abuse.

2. Correct Answer: C

Individuals suffering from bulimia nervosa follow a routine of secretive, uncontrolled or binge eating (ingesting an abnormally large amount of food within a set period of time) followed by behaviors to rid the body of the food consumed. This includes self-induced vomiting and/or the misuse of laxatives, diet pills, diuretics (water pills), excessive exercise, or fasting. Bulimia afflicts approximately 1 to 3% of adolescents in the US, and the illness usually begins in late adolescence or early adult life.

3. Correct Answer: A

Anxiety or obsessive compulsive disorder (OCD) can look like ADHD. Drug abuse, especially when it occurs in the school setting, can also make an individual appear inattentive and impulsive. It may be wise to perform a drug screen on some adults and adolescents who present with symptoms of inattention, irritability and impulsivity. Onset of symptoms may help differentiate ADHD from some other disorders. ADHD generally begins before the age of 7.

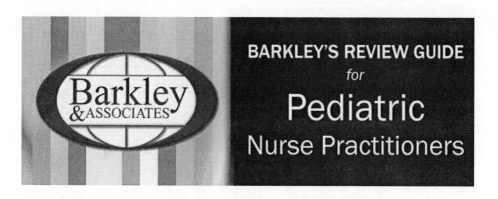
Cardiovascular Issues and Disorders

Blood Flow Through the Heart

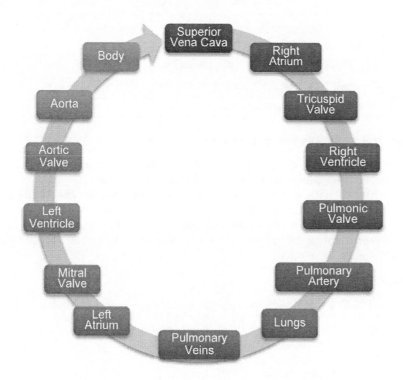

Heart Sounds and Anatomical Location	
S1	Mitral/tricuspid (AV) valves closure
S2	Aortic/pulmonic (semilunar) valves closure
Systole	Period between S1 and S2
Diastole	Period between S2 and S1
S3	"Ken-tuck'-y"; increased fluid states
S4	"Ten-ne-ssee"; stiff ventricular wall

Auscultatory Areas	
Aortic	Second right ICS
Pulmonic	Second left ICS
Erb's point	Third left ICS, sternal border
Tricuspid	Fifth ICS (sternal border)
Mitral	Fifth ICS (near nipple line)

Congenital Heart Diseases/Defects

1. These are a variety of cardiovascular malformations resulting from abnormal structural development in the first trimester
2. The etiology is multifactorial and includes chromosomal abnormalities, adverse environmental conditions and unknown factors
3. Overall, congenital heart disease occurs in 8:1,000 births
4. Ventricular septal defect (VSD) comprises up to 30% of all congenital heart defects

Congenital Heart Defects

1. Congenital
   a. Acyanotic lesions (left to right shunting)
   b. Cyanotic lesions (right to left shunting)
   c. Obstructive lesions
2. Acquired:
   a. Hypertension
   b. Rheumatic heart disease
   c. Kawasaki disease
   d. Congestive heart failure (CHF)

Acyanotic Defects (left to right shunting)

1. Atrial septal defect (ASD)

      a.   Wide, fixed S2
      b.   Grade II to III/VI systolic ejection murmur
      c.   Heard best at the left upper sternal border (LUSB)
      d.   May have mid-diastolic rumble at LUSB
      e.   ECG findings:
            i.   Small ASD: Normal
            ii.   Hemodynamically significant: Right axis deviation and mild right ventricular hypertrophy (RVH) or bundle branch block in V1
      f.   X-ray: May show cardiomegaly with increased pulmonary vascular markings if hemodynamically significant lesion

2.   Ventricular septal defect (VSD)
      a.   30% of all congenital heart defects
      b.   II to V/VI holosystolic murmur, loudest at the left lower sternal border (LLSB)
      c.   A systolic thrill may be felt at the LLSB
      d.   S2 may be narrow
      e.   ECG findings:
            i.   Small VSD: Normal
            ii.   Medium VSD: Left ventricular hypertrophy + left atrial enlargement
            iii.   Large VSD: Biventricular hypertrophy + left atrial enlargement and RVH
      f.   X-ray: May show cardiomegaly and increased pulmonary vascular markings depending on the amount of left to right shunting

3.   Atrioventricular septal defect (AVSD)
      a.   Same/similar findings as ASD
      b.   5% of all congenital heart defects
      c.   Higher incidence amongst Down syndrome children
      d.   Surgery is immediately indicated if refractory to management or when failure to thrive is present, generally before 1 year of age

4.   Patent ductus arteriosis (PDA)
      a.   5% to 10% of congenital heart defects in term infants
      b.   40% to 60% of congenital heart defects in preterm infants weighing < 1,500 g
      c.   II to IV/VI holosystolic murmur
      d.   "Machinery" quality murmur loudest at the LUSB
      e.   ECG findings:
            i.   Small PDA: Normal or left ventricular hypertrophy (LVH)
            ii.   Large PDA: Biventricular hypertrophy
      f.   X-ray findings: May have cardiomegaly and increased pulmonary vascular markings depending on the size of the shunt

Cyanotic Defects (right to left shunting)

1. Transposition of the great arteries
    a. Sharp S1
    b. Loud single or narrow split S2
    c. Occurs in the newborn period
    d. Associated with closure of the PDA
    e. Incidence: 8% of congenital heart defects
    f. Extreme cyanosis
    g. May have murmur from associated VSD or pulmonic stenosis (PS)
    h. ECG findings: May see right axis deviation and RVH
    i. X-ray: "Egg on a string" with cardiomegaly; may also have increased pulmonary vascular markings
2. Tetralogy of Fallot
    a. Four defects:
        i. Large VSD
        ii. Pulmonary stenosis
        iii. Overriding aorta
        iv. RVH
    b. Loud systolic ejection murmur at the middle and upper left sternal border (M-LUSB)
    c. A thrill may be present
    d. ECG findings: Right axis deviation and right ventricular hypertrophy
    e. X-ray findings: Boot-shaped heart with normal size + pulmonary vascular markings
3. Tricuspid atresia
    a. Absent tricuspid valve and hypoplastic right ventricle and pulmonary artery
    b. Must have PDA, VSD or ASD for survival (septal/ductal dependent)
    c. Single S2
    d. II to III/VI systolic regurgitation murmur at the LLSB with a VSD
    e. ECG findings: Superior QRS axis, right atrial enlargement, and LVH
    f. X-ray findings: Normal size heart or slightly enlarged; may be boot-shaped
4. Truncus arteriosis
    a. Loud, S2 with mid-diastolic murmur
    b. Failure of arteries to divide
    c. Incidence: Rare; about 0.4% of congenital heart defects
    d. Presents in the neonatal period
5. Pulmonary atresia
    a. Occurs in 1:10,000 live births
    b. No pulmonary valve exists

    c.   The right ventricle acts as a blind pouch that may be underdeveloped or small

    d.   The tricuspid valve is often poorly-developed

    e.   Cyanosis occurs upon closure of the PDA

Obstructive Lesions

1.   Aortic stenosis
    a.   Systolic thrill at the right upper sternal border (RUSB)
    b.   Ejection click present which does not vary with respirations
    c.   Harsh systolic ejection murmur, grade II to IV/VI at the second right ICS or third left ICS radiates to the neck and apex
    d.   Narrow pulse pressure is present if stenosis is severe
    e.   ECG findings:
        i.   Mild: Normal
        ii.   Moderate-severe: Left ventricular hypertrophy (LVH)
    f.   X-ray findings: Usually normal
    g.   If severe, may present with CHF in the first year of life

2.   Pulmonic stenosis
    a.   Systolic murmur loudest at the LUSB; grade II to V/VI ejection click at the LUSB with valvular pulmonary stenosis
    b.   Intensity of click decreases with inspiration and increases with expiration
    c.   Thrill at the LUSB radiating to the back and sides
    d.   Incidence: 7% of all congenital heart defects
    e.   20% are associated with other defects
    f.   ECG findings:
        i.   Mild: Normal
        ii.   Moderate: Right axis deviation and RVH
        iii.   Severe: Right atrial enlargement and right ventricular enlargement with strain
    g.   X-ray findings: Usually normal size with normal or decreased pulmonary vascular markings

3.   Coarctation of the aorta
    a.   8% to 10% of congenital heart defects
    b.   Male to female ratio: 2:1
    c.   May present in infancy as CHF, in children with hypertension, or a murmur
    d.   II to III/VI systolic ejection murmur with radiation to the left interscapular area
    e.   May have an ejection click at the apex and RUSB if the bicuspid valve is involved
    f.   BP in lower extremities will be lower than in upper extremities
    g.   Pulse oximetry discrepancy of > 5% between the upper and lower extremities

h. ECG findings:
 i. In infancy: RVH or right bundle branch block
 ii. In older children: Left ventricular hypertrophy (LVH)
 iii. X-ray findings: Cardiomegaly, pulmonary venous congestion; rib notching due to collateral circulation is seen in children > 5 years of age, but not in infants

Common Genetic Syndromes and Associated Cardiac Defects

1. DiGeorge syndrome: Aortic arch anomalies
2. Trisomies:
 a. Trisomy 18/Edward's
 b. Trisomy XXI/Down syndrome: Atrioventricular septal defects, VSD
3. Marfan syndrome: Aortic regurgitation, mitral valve prolapse
4. Turner syndrome: Coarcation of the aorta, tricuspid aortic valve

Signs/Symptoms

1. Prenatal, birth and family history are critically important
2. Assess for history of:
 a. Frequent respiratory infections
 b. Exercise intolerance
 c. Color changes
 d. Tachypnea during sleep
 e. Feeding problems
 f. Diaphoresis
3. Heart sounds
 a. ASD: Systolic ejection at LUSB; may also hear split S2
 b. VSD: Loud holosystolic murmur at the LUSB; may palpate a thrill
 c. PDA: Soft systolic murmur "machinery" at LUSB
 d. Transposition of Great Arteries (TGA): Sharp S1, loud single or narrow split S2
 e. Tetralogy of Fallot (TOF): Loud harsh systolic ejection murmur with thrill; may also see a right ventricular heave
 f. Tricuspid atresia: Loud S1, crescendo-decrescendo holosystolic murmur
 g. Truncus arteriosis: Loud S2, mid-diastolic murmur, may be other regurgitant and mid sternal high pitched diastolic murmurs present
 h. Aortic stenosis: Systolic murmur loudest at RUSB
 i. Pulmonic stenosis: Systolic murmur loudest at LUSB
 j. Coarctation of the aorta (COA): Soft bruit at LUSB
4. Other signs of individual disorders include cyanosis, chest heaves, palpable thrills, and disequal pulses
5. Abnormal respiratory patterns
6. Edema in older children

7. Clubbing
8. Cyanosis: Central or peripheral
9. Beck's triad:
    a. Lowered BP; narrowing pulse pressure
    b. Distant/muffled heart sounds
    c. Jugular venous distention

Management

1. Referral to pediatric cardiologist
2. Ensure optimal primary care and anticipatory guidance

Innocent Murmurs

Murmurs found in childhood that do not signify any pathology

1. No associated symptoms, failure to thrive, or cyanosis
2. Also known as functional, benign, or physiologic
3. Occurs in > 50% of children
4. Routine testing is not indicated; referral only required if suspicion of pathology exists

Still's Murmur

1. Most common innocent murmur
2. Musical systolic murmur
3. Heard best between LLSB and apex
4. Due to turbulence in the left ventricular outflow tract

Pulmonary Flow Murmur

1. Systolic ejection murmur
2. Heard best at the second ICS left sternal border
3. Due to turbulent flow in right ventricular outflow tract

Supraclavicular Arterial Bruit

1. Early systolic murmur
2. Heard above clavicles
3. Caused by turbulence at the branching of the brachiocephalic arteries

Physiologic Peripheral Pulmonary Stenosis

1. Low intensity systolic murmur
2. Heard best at LUSB, axillae, and posterior thorax to 6 months of age
3. Caused by hypoplasia of the branch of the pulmonary artery

Venous Hum

1. Continuous humming murmur
2. RUSB

3.   Heard best in the sitting position; disappears in the supine position

Hypertension

A persistent elevation of average systolic/diastolic blood pressure $\geq 95^{th}$ percentile for age and sex with measurements obtained on at least three separate occasions

1.   Prevalence is low; approximately 1 to 3% in children

Definitions of Pediatric Hypertension

1.   < 2 years: > 112/74
2.   3 to 5 years: > 116/76
3.   6 to 9 years: > 122/78
4.   10 to 12 years: > 126/82
5.   13 to 15 years: > 136/86
6.   16 years: > 142/92, no report

Theories of Primary Hypertension

1.   Central nervous system (CNS) hyperactivity
2.   Renin-angiotensin system
3.   Defect in natriuresis
4.   Elevated intracellular Na+ and Ca++

Signs/Symptoms

1.   Often there are none
2.   Headaches
3.   Visual Problems
4.   Dizziness
5.   Respiratory distress
6.   Irritability
7.   Nosebleed
8.   More commonly recognized in adolescents

Causes of Secondary Hypertension

1.   Coarctation of aorta
2.   Renal disease
3.   Renal vascular disease
4.   Hyperaldosteronism and Cushing's syndrome
5.   Pheochromocytoma
6.   Neurogenic tumors

Physical Exam Findings

1.   Most significant is the elevated blood pressures identified in the definition
2.   A loud aortic second heart sound and early systolic ejection click may occur
3.   S4 due to decreased left ventricle compliance is common

4.	Peripheral pulses may be abnormal in some secondary cases
5.	Retinal changes on ophthalmic exam may be noted in advanced chronic cases
6.	In secondary hypertension, findings are consistent with the underlying disorder

Laboratory/Diagnostic Findings

1.	In uncomplicated essential hypertension, laboratory findings are usually normal
2.	Common considerations for secondary hypertension:
	a.	CT scan for suspected renovascular disease
	b.	Chest x-ray to rule out coarctation of the aorta or cardiomegaly
	c.	Plasma aldosterone level to rule out aldosteronism
	d.	Morning and evening cortisol levels to rule out Cushing's syndrome

Management (Baseline Studies)

1.	UA, basic metabolic panel (BMP), CBC, calcium, phosphorous, uric acid, cholesterol, and triglycerides
2.	ECG for dysrhythmias, bundle branch block, or LVH
3.	PA and lateral chest x-rays

Management (Non-pharmacologic)

1.	Weight reduction
2.	Low sodium diet (decrease salt intake to at least 80 to 100 mEq/day)
3.	Cessation of smoking
4.	Avoidance/reduction of alcohol intake
5.	Stress management
6.	Relaxation and exercise; aerobic exercise (especially for adolescents)
7.	Referral to a cardiologist

Rheumatic Fever/Heart Disease

A post-infectious inflammatory disease that can affect the heart, joints and CNS

1.	Rheumatic fever usually follows a group A strep infection of the upper respiratory tract and is most common in ages 6 to 15
2.	The most common affected valve is the mitral

Signs/Symptoms

1.	Diagnosis of an initial attack of rheumatic fever plus 2 major or 1 major and 2 minor Jones' criteria:
	a.	Major manifestations:
		i.	Carditis
		ii.	Polyarthritis

    iii. Chorea
    iv. Erythema marginatum
    v. Subcutaneous nodules
  b. Minor criteria:
    i. Arthralgia without objective inflammation
    ii. Fever > 102.2°F (39°C)
    iii. Elevated levels of acute phase reactants [i.e., erythrocyte sedimentation rate (ESR) and C-reactive protein]
    iv. Prolonged PR interval on ECG with evidence of a group A β-hemolytic *Streptococcus* infection
2. Findings based on manifestations

Laboratory/Diagnostics

1. Acute phase reactants:
  a. Positive throat culture
  b. Positive rapid strep culture
  c. Increased or rising strep antibody titer
2. ECG
3. Echocardiogram

Management

1. Refer to a pediatric cardiologist
2. Aggressive management of the strep infection
3. Bed rest if acute carditis is present
4. Symptomatic treatment of arthritis or carditis
5. Prophylactic antibiotics for invasive procedures, as indicated

Kawasaki Disease

Acute febrile syndrome causing vasculitis

1. The leading cause of coronary artery disease in children of an infectious etiology
2. Most commonly noted in children under the age of 2
3. Occurs most commonly in children of Asian ethnicity

Signs/Symptoms

1. Persistent fever for > 5 days
2. Red eyes, tongue, and/or throat
3. Erythema
4. Edema of hands and/or feet
5. Vomiting and diarrhea
6. Abdominal pain
7. Dry, peeling skin
8. Joint pain

9. Bilateral conjunctival injection
10. Lymphadenopathy
11. Arthritis and arthralgias
12. Tachycardia

Diagnostic Criteria

The patient must have a fever, as well as 4 of the criteria listed below; if the patient has more than 4 of the criteria, coronary vessel involvement is most likely

1. Fever for $\geq$ 5 days
2. Bilateral conjunctival injection without exudate
3. Polymorphous rash (urticarial or pruritic)
4. Inflammatory changes of the lips and oral cavity
5. Changes in extremities (e.g., erythema, edema, etc.)
6. Cervical lymphadenopathy

Laboratory/Diagnostics

1. None specific
2. Thrombocytosis
3. Leukocytosis
4. Elevated erythrocyte sedimentation rate (ESR)
5. Positive C-reactive protein
6. ECG changes in approximately 30% of patients
   a. ST segment changes
   b. Decreased R wave voltage
   c. Prolonged PR or QT interval
   d. Dysrhythmias

Management

1. Immediate referral to a physician
2. Intravenous gamma globulin, as appropriate
   a. No live virus vaccines for at least five months after gamma globulin
3. High dose ASA

Heart Failure

A syndrome that results when cardiac output is insufficient to meet the metabolic needs of the body

1. Heart failure may be the result of a congenital defect as discussed previously or acquired as a result of myocarditis, rheumatic disease, or cardiomyopathy

Signs/Symptoms

1. Increased respiratory rate

2. Poor feeding
3. Decreased exercise tolerance
4. Chronic cough
5. Tachycardia
6. Hepatosplenomegaly
7. Pallor or mottling
8. Puffy eyelids
9. Weakly palpable peripheral pulses
10. Wheezing or adventitious

Laboratory/Diagnostic Findings

1. Echocardiogram will show wall motion, valve function, and estimate ejection fraction
2. ECG may show deviation or the underlying problem
3. Chest radiograph: To reveal cardiomegaly, vascular congestion, etc.

Management

1. Refer to a cardiology specialist
2. Inotropes (e.g., Digoxin to increase the contractility)
3. Diuretics
4. Afterload reducing agents (i.e., antihypertensives)

Sample Questions

1.   A 2-year-old comes into the clinic with a 4-day history of fever, erythema of the palms and soles, strawberry tongue, and erythmatous cracked lips. In addition, her cervical lymph nodes are palpated and 2 cm in diameter. What is the most likely diagnosis based on the history and physical exam?

   a.   Rheumatic fever
   b.   Group A β-hemolytic streptococcus infection
   c.   Kawasaki disease
   d.   Scarlet fever

2.   During a routine pediatric physical exam, you hear a cardiac murmur. Which of the following requires referral to a cardiologist at this time?

   a.   A 4-year-old with a grade 5 murmur heard best on right side when sitting up and head turned away; it disappears in a supine position
   b.   A 2-year-old with a grade 2 systolic murmur with a musical sound heard at the lower left sternal border extending to apex; it is loudest in supine position and decreases upon sitting or standing
   c.   A 14-year-old with a grade 3 systolic ejection murmur heard best at the left sternal border in the second and third intercostal spaces; the murmur increases with expiration and decreases with inspiration, sitting, or standing
   d.   A 1-year-old with a grade 2 harsh mid to late systolic ejection murmur at the upper left sternal border with radiation throughout and an intermittent systolic ejection click

3.   When counseling the parents of an infant with congestive heart failure (CHF) about feeding, you should know that the infant has a need for:

   a.   Increased fluids
   b.   Increased calories
   c.   Decreased fats
   d.   Decreased protein

Answers

1. Correct Answer: C

Rheumatic fever includes red swollen painful joints pain, tachycardia out of proportion to fever, rash-erythema marginatum, and chorea. Patients with group A β-*hemolytic streptococcus* infection may have fever, but it might not be as prolonged. A strawberry tongue may be present, and cracked lips are possible. However, the lips, hands, and soles would not be red. Scarlet fever starts with a white, furry tongue but would turn to a red strawberry tongue by the 4th day. Scarlet fever would also present with enlarged tonsils and a pinpoint erythematous dry rash that blanches on pressure located on the trunk and skinfolds. Kawasaki disease is characterized by fever 4 to 5 days, erythema of the palms and soles, edema of hands and feet, polymorphous exanthema, and cervical lymphadenopathy more than 1.5 cm.

2. Correct Answer: D

Choice A represents a venous hum, B is a Still's murmur, and C is a pulmonary flow murmur. Choices A, B and C are all innocent murmurs. Choice D is indicative of pulmonic stenosis and requires a referral for confirmation and treatment and is the correct answer.

3. Correct Answer: B

The diet should also include increased protein and increased fat to facilitate the child's intake of sufficient calories. Fluids must be carefully monitored because of the CHF. The diet should include increased protein and increased fat to facilitate the child's intake of sufficient calories. The metabolic rate of infants with CHF is greater because of poor cardiac function and increased heart and respiratory rates. Infants' caloric needs are greater than those of average infants, yet their ability to take in calories is diminished by their fatigue.

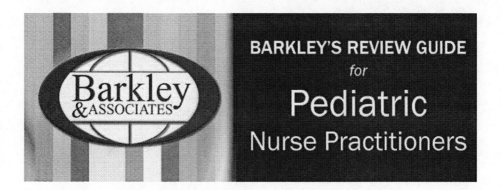

Gastrointestinal Issues and Disorders

Gastroenteritis

A nonspecific term applied to a syndrome of acute nausea, vomiting and diarrhea as the result of an acute irritation/inflammation of the gastric mucosa

1.   Children attending day care are at increased risk

Causes/Incidence

1.   Viruses are the majority of causes that are especially active during the winter
        a.   Rotovirus is 50% of viral cases
        b.   Adenovirus
2.   Bacterial
        a.   *Salmonella*
        b.   *Campylobacteria* (odorous stool)
        c.   *Shigella* (fever spikes, bloody stools, febrile seizures)
        d.   *E. Coli* (mild loose stools)
3.   Parasitic
4.   Inorganic food contents
5.   Emotional stress

Signs/Symptoms

1.   Nausea
2.   Vomiting
3.   Hyperactive bowel sounds
4.   Watery diarrhea
5.   General "sick" feeling (fever when septic)
6.   Anorexia
7.   Crampy abdominal pain and/or abdominal distention

Incubation Periods

Organism	Incubation
E. Coli	24 to 72 hours
Campylobacter	2 to 5 days
Staphylococcus	1 to 6 hours
Shigella/Salmonella	8 to 24 hours
Botulism	12 to 36 hours
Giardia	7 to 21 days

Physical Exam Findings

1. Fever is variable
2. Tachycardia
3. Dehydration may be evident

Assessment of Dehydration

Variable	Mild (3% to 5%)	Moderate (6% to 9%)	Severe (≥10%)
Blood Pressure	Normal	Normal	Normal, decreased
Pulse/Heart Rate	Normal	Increased	Severe, decreased
CAP Refill	WNL	WNL	Prolonged (> 3 seconds)
Skin turgor	Normal	Decreased	Decreased
Fontanel	Normal	Sunken (slightly)	Sunken
Urine	Slightly decreased	< 1mg/kg/hour	< 1mg/kg/hour

Diagnostic Tests/Findings

1. None indicated unless symptoms persist more than 72 hours or bloody stool is present
2. Stool guaiac may be positive with bacterial infections
3. Stool for white blood cells
4. Stool culture
5. Stool for ova and parasites test

Management

Daycare exclusion: Rotavirus, *E. Coli* and *Shigella*; only *E. Coli* and *Shigella* require 2 negative stool cultures prior to return to daycare

1.   Frequent supportive therapy is often all that is needed:
   a.   Oral rehydration therapy (ORT) with appropriate rehydration solution in mild to moderately dehydrated patients
      i.   Assessing fluid deficit is based on pre-illness weight, calculated as follows:
         1.   Fluid deficit (L) formula: Pre-illness weight (kg) − Illness weight (kg)
         2.   Percentage dehydration formula: [(Pre-illness weight − Illness weight)/Pre-illness weight] × 100% Pre-illness weight
   b.   Mild dehydration: 50 mL/kg oral rehydration solution over 4 hours
   c.   Moderate dehydration: 100mL/kg oral rehydration solution over 4 hours
   d.   Do not give the following as oral rehydration fluids: Undiluted juices (apple or orange), Coca-Cola, Gatorade, ginger ale, or milk due to potential hyperosmolar effects
   e.   Breastfeeding should continue
   f.   Formula-fed infants should continue their regular formula
   g.   Foods to encourage:
      i.   Complex carbohydrates such as the **BRAT** diet (**b**ananas, **r**ice, **a**pple sauce, **t**oast), baked potatoes, noodles, crackers, and cereals that are not high in simple sugars
      ii.   Soups (clear broths with rice, noodles, or vegetables)
      iii.   Yogurt, vegetables (without butter), fresh fruits (though not canned in syrup)
   h.   Foods to minimize:
      i.   Those high in fat or simple sugars (e.g., fried foods, juices, sodas)
      ii.   Plain or tap water should not be the only source of oral fluid
   i.   Bed rest during the acute phase with progression as tolerated
2.   Anti-motility drugs should be used judiciously:
   a.   Not usually indicated in mild forms of disease
   b.   May prolong the illness
   c.   Should not be used in patients with fever and/or bloody stools
3.   Antibiotic therapy
   a.   Indicated when an organism (except *Salmonella*) is isolated and symptoms are not resolved
   b.   Considered when the patient experiences more than 8 to 10 stools daily
   c.   Considered when the patient is immunocompromised
   d.   Indicated when leukocytes or dysentery are present
   e.   Specific organisms:
      i.   *Salmonella*

1. If an infant is more than 6 months old, toxicity or immune-compromised: Cefotaxime or ceftriaxone for 10 to 14 days
2. Antibiotics are not usually necessary unless the infection spreads from the intestines: Then, treat with ampicillin, gentamicin, trimethoprim/ sulfamethoxazole (TMP/SMZ) or ciprofloxacin
    ii. *Shigella*
    Antibiotics (trimethoprim/sulfamethoxazole, alternate: cefixime for 5 days)
    iii. *E. Coli*
    Usually self-limiting; duration shortened by TMP/SMZ
    iv. *Yersinia*
    TMP/SMX, aminoglycosides, cefotaxime, tetracycline (for patients > 8 years old); only treat when bacteremia or extra-intestinal infections are present or if the patient is immunocompromised
    v. Giardia
    Metronidiazole is the drug of choice
4. Prophylaxis
    Traveler's diarrhea prophylaxis (Bismuth subsalicylate)
    a. Prevention is the best treatment:
        i. Cook ground meat and chicken thoroughly
        ii. Cook food until it is not runny
        iii. Cooking surface cleansing (e.g., cutting boards)
        iv. Teach hand washing

Gastroesophageal Reflux Disease (GERD)

A condition in which gastric contents pass into the esophagus from the stomach through the lower esophageal sphincter (LES)

1. The 3 classes of gastroesophageal reflux disease (GERD) are:
    a. Physiological: Infrequent, episodic vomiting
    b. Functional: Painless, effortless vomiting with no physical sequelae
    c. Pathological: Frequent vomiting with alteration in physical functioning such as failure to thrive (FTT) and aspiration pneumonia
2. The etiology is unclear, possibly multifactorial in origin
3. 85% of premature infants and more than 70% of infants weighing less than 1700 g have pathological GERD; 40% have symptomatic improvement by 3 months of age and 70% are symptom-free by 18 months

Signs/Symptoms

1.   Choking
2.   Coughing/wheezing
3.   Weight loss
4.   Irritability
5.   Dysphagia
6.   Recurrent vomiting
7.   Heartburn
8.   Painful belching/abdominal pain
9.   Stool pattern changes
10. Other: Sore throat, pharyngitis, otis media, dental erosions

Laboratory/Diagnostics

1.   Complete blood count with differential to rule out anemia and infections
2.   Urinalysis and urine culture
3.   Stool for occult blood
4.   Abdominal ultrasonography to rule out pyloric stenosis (if age appropriate)
5.   Esophageal pH monitoring, with a pH lower than 4 indicating reflux (refer to a gastroenterologist)
6.   Endoscopy to rule out esophagitis if indicated (gastroenterologist)

Management

1.   Small frequent feedings:
     a.   Burp frequently during feeding
     b.   Continue breastfeeding
     c.   Avoid formula changes
     d.   One tablespoon of rice cereal per ounce of formula
     e.   Elevate head after feeding
2.   For older children, avoid chocolate, caffeine, high-fat foods, spicy foods, alcohol, and bed-time snacks
3.   Medications:
     a.   Histamine H2-receptor antagonists to inhibit gastric acid secretion caused by histamine [e.g., famotidine (Pepcid AC), ranitidine (Zantac)]
     b.   Proton pump inhibitors (PPIs) to block gastric acid secretion caused by histamine, acetylcholine, or gastrin [e.g., omeprazole (Pilosec)]
     c.   Metoclopramide (Reglan) to hasten gastric emptying (note, the Food and Drug Administration's Black Box warning for tardive dyskinesia)
4.   Follow-up frequently to monitor growth parameters; parent education
5.   Consider referral to GI specialist

Pyloric Stenosis

Obstruction resulting from thickening of the circular muscle of the pylorus, occurring in 1:500 infants

1. Cause is unclear; may be familial predisposition
2. Males more often affected
3. Most common in Caucasians
4. Breast feeding delays presentation

Signs/Symptoms

1. Presentation is usually from 3 weeks to 4 months of age
2. Projectile non-bilious vomiting after eating
3. Hungry after vomiting
4. Poor weight gain or weight loss
5. Eventually becomes dehydrated
6. Visible peristaltic waves
7. Palpable mass (pyloric olive) after vomiting

Laboratory/Diagnostics

1. Abdominal ultrasound
2. Upper gastrointestinal (GI) if ultrasound is not diagnostic: Commonly shows "string sign" (narrowed pyloric channel)

Management

1. Surgical referral; prognosis excellent

Intussusception

Acute prolapse (telescoping) of one part of the intestine into another adjacent segment of the intestine

1. Cause is unknown, but may be due to adenovirus
2. Other proposed causes include celiac disease, cystic fibrosis
3. More common in males
4. Most cases occur before age 2 years

Signs/Symptoms

1. Previously healthy infant develops acute colicky pain
2. Non-bilious vomiting
3. Progressive lethargy
4. Current jelly stool: Late presentation
5. Sausage shaped mass in right upper quadrant
6. Progressive distention/tenderness
7. If not reduced, perforation and shock may occur

Mneumonic for Intussusception in Infants: ABCDEF

A = Abdominal or anal sausage (mass)
B = Blood from rectum (currant jelly)
C = Colic: Draw up legs
D = Distention, dehydration, shock
E = Emesis
F = Face pale

Laboratory/Diagnostics

1.   Radiograph to clarify diagnosis
2.   Barium enema: Diagnostic and produces reduction

Management

1.   Barium reduction as above
2.   May require emergency surgery
3.   Fatal if not treated urgently

Appendicitis

Inflammation of the appendix, precipitated by obstruction due to feces, a foreign body, inflammation, or neoplasm

1.   If untreated, gangrene and perforation may develop within 36 hours

Causes/Incidence

1.   Most common in males 10 to 30 years old
2.   Affects approximately 10% of the population

Signs/Symptoms

1.   Begins with vague, colicky umbilical pain
2.   After several hours, pain shifts to right lower quadrant abdominal pain (RLQ)
3.   RLQ guarding with rebound tenderness
4.   Psoas sign: Pain with right thigh extension
5.   Obturator sign: Pain with internal rotation of the right thigh
6.   Local abdominal tenderness
7.   Pain worsened and localized with cough
8.   Nausea with 1 to 2 episodes of vomiting (more vomiting suggests another diagnosis)
9.   Sense of constipation; infrequently diarrhea
10.   Fever (low grade)

Laboratory/Diagnostics

1.   White blood cells (WBCs) 10,000 to 20,000/uL; Sedimentation rate elevated
2.   Computed tomography (CT) or ultrasound is diagnostic

Management

1.   Surgical treatment: Wound healing. Prognosis typically very good
2.   Pain management

Malabsorption

Impaired intestinal absorption of essential nutrients and electrolytes caused by enzymatic deficiencies (e.g, cystic fibrosis), infectious agents, and abnormalities of the intestinal mucosa

1.   Celiac disease (sprue) is an uncommon cause; gluten intolerance

Signs/Symptoms

1.   Failure to thrive
2.   Severe, chronic diarrhea
3.   Bulky, foul stool
4.   Vomiting
5.   Abdominal pain
6.   Protuberant abdomen
7.   Associated with vitamin deficiency or malabsorption:
      a.   Pallor
      b.   Fatigue
      c.   Hair and dermatological abnormalities
      d.   Cheilosis
      e.   Peripheral neuropathy

Laboratory/Diagnostics

1.   Stool for culture and microscopic
2.   Hemoccult: Eval mucosal damage, inflammatory disease
3.   Ova and parasite exam (O&P)
4.   Serum calcium, phosphorus, alkaline phosphatase, total protein, ferritin, folate, and liver function tests
5.   Bone age
6.   Lactose and sucrose breath hydrogen testing
7.   Sweat test if clinical suspicion of cystic fibrosis

Differential Diagnosis

1.   Failure to thrive
2.   Short stature

3. Cystic fibrosis
4. Immune deficiency
5. Hepatic disease
6. Inflammatory bowel disease
7. Chronic diarrhea/ Celiac disease

Management

1. Treat persistent enteric infections
2. Avoid offending foods: If malabsorption is a primary problem, life-time avoidance of offending foods is necessary; if malabsorption is a secondary problem, retrial of the food at intervals can be attempted
3. Refer to gastroenterology
4. Celiac disease: No wheat, oats, rye, barley
5. Cystic fibrosis: Pancreatic enzyme replacement

Hepatitis

An inflammation of the liver with resultant liver dysfunction

1. Manifestation of symptoms may be either mild and self-limiting or profound and life threatening
2. Caused by any variety of viral subtypes (hepatitis A, B, C, D, E, & G); the most common types are A, B, and C

Hepatitis A

An enteral virus, transmitted via the oral-fecal route

1. Common source outbreaks result from contaminated water and food
2. Shellfish such as raw oysters, clams, and mussels, are a frequent source of infection
3. Symptoms manifest 2 to 6 weeks after infection
4. Blood and stools are infectious during the 2 to 6 week incubation period
5. Most children are anicteric, so infections frequently go unnoticed
6. A chronic carrier state does not exist, mortality rate is very low, and fulminant hepatitis A is rare

Hepatitis B

A blood-borne virus present in saliva, semen, vaginal secretions, and all body fluids

1. Transmitted via blood and blood products, sexual activity, and mother to fetus
2. Incubation is 6 weeks to 6 months
3. Clinical features of A and B are similar, but B tends to have a more insidious onset
4. The younger the child, the greater the chance of developing a chronic state

5.   Risk of fulminant hepatitis is < 1%, but when it occurs, mortality is approximately 60%

Hepatitis C

A blood borne virus in which the source of infection is uncertain

1.   Hepatitis C accounts for 20 to 40% of all viral hepatitis
2.   Traditionally associated with blood transfusion
3.   50% of cases are related to IV drug use
4.   The risk of sexual transmission is small and maternal-neonatal transmission is rare
5.   Incubation period is variable, ranging from about 4 to 12 weeks
6.   Most affected children are anicteric

Hepatitis Signs/Symptoms

1.   Pre-icteric: Fatigue, malaise, anorexia, n/v, headache, aversion to smoking and alcohol
2.   Icteric: Weight loss, jaundice, pruritus, right upper quadrant abdominal pain (RUQ pain), clay colored stool, dark urine
3.   Physical appearance depends on the level of virulence and type of virus; may range from mildly ill to very toxic
4.   Low grade fever may be present
5.   Hepatosplenomegaly may be present
6.   Diffuse abdominal pain, tenderness over the liver area
7.   Dark urine and light-colored stool

Laboratory/Diagnostics

1.   WBC low to normal
2.   Urinalysis (UA): Proteinuria, bilirubinuria
3.   Elevated aminotransferase (AST) and aminotranferease (ALT) (500 to 2,000 IU/L)
4.   AST and ALT rise prior to onset of jaundice; will fall after jaundice presents
5.   Lactate dehydrogenase (LDH), bilirubin, alkaline phosphate, prothrombin time test (PT) are normal or slightly elevated

<u>Serology tests depend on the type of hepatitis</u>

Virus	Serology
Active hepatitis A	Anti-HAV, IgM
Recovered hepatitis A	Anti-HAV, IgG
Active hepatitis B	HBsAg, HBeAg, Anti-HBc, IgM
Chronic hepatitis B	HBsAg, Anti-HBc, Anti-Hbe, IgM, IgG
Recovered hepatitis B	Anti-HBc, Anti-HBsAg
Acute hepatitis C	Anti-HCV, HCV RNA
Chronic hepatitis C	Anti-HCV, HCV RNA

Management

1. Generally supportive: Rest during the active phase
2. Increase fluids to 3,000 to 4,000 millilters/day
3. Vitamin K for prolonged PT (> 15 sec)
4. Avoid alcohol and medications detoxified by the liver
5. No or low protein diet
6. Rebetron (interferon and ribavirin) may be prescribed for hepatitis C
7. Patient education
8. Hepatitis B immune globulin (passive immunization) is recommended for infants born to known hepatitis B surface antigen (HbsAg)-positive mothers
9. Hepatitis B immunization
   a. Hepatitis B vaccine given in 3 doses (at birth, 1 month, and 6 months)
   b. Patients who are unresponsive can receive up to three additional doses at 1 to 2 month intervals with serologic testing after each dose

Sample Questions

1. A 6-month-old female presents to the emergency department with a one-day history of vomiting and diarrhea. The infant has normal vital signs, capillary refill is less than two seconds, and is generally happy in her mother's arms. The mother reports slightly decreased urine output since this morning. Based on this information, management of this infant should include:

    a. Administration of normal saline bolus of 20ml/kg
    b. Encouragement of infant formula as tolerated and further monitoring
    c. Administration of 1 dose of an anti-motility drug and continuation of clear liquids
    d. Give 50ml/kg of liquid of choice over 8 hours

2. A 2-month-old male presents to the emergency department with a history of irritability, persistent stuffy nose, recurrent vomiting, and failure to thrive. The most likely cause is:

    a. Pyloric stenosis
    b. Meningitis
    c. Protein allergy to formula
    d. GERD

3. Gastroenteritis is a condition that causes irritation and inflammation of the stomach and intestines and the usual symptoms are:

    a. Diarrhea, crampy abdominal pain, nausea, and vomiting
    b. Weakness, lethargy, nausea and vomiting
    c. High fever, crampy abdominal pain, nausea, and vomiting
    d. Severe dehydration along with nausea, and vomiting

Answers

1. Correct Answer: B

In mild dehydration, oral rehydration is indicated. Formula fed infants should continue with their regular formula. Avoid fruit juices, Gatorade, milk, and liquids high in sugar content. Rehydration should include 50ml/kg of appropriate oral rehydration solution over 4 hours.

2. Correct Answer: D

These are the signs and symptoms of GERD.

3. Correct Answer: A

Gastroenteritis is a condition that causes irritation and inflammation of the stomach and the gastrointestinal tract. Diarrhea, crampy abdominal pain, nausea, and vomiting are the most common symptoms.

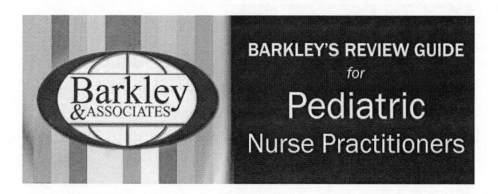

Dermatological and Communicable Issues and Disorders

Evaluation of Skin Disorders

A systematic approach to the evaluation of skin disorders is to identify the morphology, configuration, and distribution

Morphology

The character of the lesion itself

1. Macule: A flat discoloration
2. Patch: A flat discoloration that looks as though it is a collection of multiple, tiny pigment changes; may be some subtle surface change
3. Papule: A small (< 0.5 cm), elevated, firm skin lesion
4. Nodule: An elevated, firm lesion > 0.5 cm
5. Tumor: A firm, elevated lump
6. Wheal: A lesion raised above the surface and extending a bit below the epidermis; many times an allergic reaction (either contact or systemic)
7. Plaque: A scaly, elevated lesion; the classic lesion of psoriasis
8. Vesicle: A small (< 0.5 cm), lesion filled with serous fluid
9. Bulla: Serous fluid-filled vesicles > 0.5 cm
10. Pustule: A small (< 0.5 cm) pus-filled lesion
11. Abscess: A pus-filled lesion > 0.5 cm
12. Cyst: Large, raised lesions filled with serous fluid, blood, and puss

Special Note

1. Primary Lesion: First appearing
2. Secondary Lesions: Follows primary lesions

Configuration

How the lesions present on the body

1. Solitary or discrete: Individual or distinct lesions that remain separate
2. Grouped: Linear cluster
3. Confluent: Lesions that run together
4. Linear: Scratch, streak, line, or stripe

5.   Annular: Circular , beginning in the center and spreading to the periphery
6.   Polycyclic: Annular lesions merge

Distribution

Where on the body the lesions appear

1.   Face
2.   Trunk
3.   Upper extremities
4.   Groin
5.   Dermatomal
6.   Feet
7.   Axilla

Acne

A polymorphic skin disorder characterized by comedones, papules, pustules and cysts

1.   Cause is unknown but appears to be activated by androgens in genetically predisposed individuals
2.   Can be exacerbated by steroids and anticonvulsants
3.   Food has not been demonstrated to be a contributing factor
4.   Acne is more common and severe in males

Signs/Symptoms

1.   Comedones, papules, pustules nodules and/or cysts on the face and or upper trunk
      a.   Comedones
          i.   Open: Blackheads; opening in the skin capped with blackened mass of skin debris
          ii.   Closed: Whiteheads; obstructed opening which may rupture, casing low-grade local inflammatory reaction
2.   Types of acne
      a.   Mild: Comedones present; few papules and pustules (< 10); no nodules
      b.   Moderate: Comedones (10 to 40); several to many papules and pustules (10 to 40)
      c.   Moderately severe: 40 papules and pustules; larger, deeper nodular inflamed lesions (< 5)
      d.   Severe: Presence of numerous or extensive papules and pustules; many nodular lesions
3.   Depressed or hypertrophic scars
4.   Occasionally mild discomfort from swollen lesion
5.   In women, may be exacerbated just prior to menses

Laboratory/Diagnostics

1.   None indicated, except to identify causative organism in atypical folliculitis

Management

1.   Non-pharmacologic:
        a.   Avoidance of topical, oil-based products
        b.   Use of oil-free, mild soaps, cleansers and moisturizers
2.   Pharmacologic:
        a.   In mild acne, topical treatment with benzoyl peroxide (2.5 to 10%)
                i.   If not responsive, retinoic acid (0.025% to 0.1%)
                         *pregnancy category C
                ii.   Tretinoin (Retin-A 0.1% cream)
                iii.   Tretinoin (Retin-A 0.025 gel) or microsphere (Retin-A
                         0.1% gel)
                iv.   Tretinoin is inactivated by UV light and oxidized by
                         benzoyl peroxide (should only be applied at night and not
                         used concomitantly with benzoyl peroxide)
        b.   Salicylic acid preparations (e.g., Neutrogena 2% wash, etc.)
        c.   Topical antibiotics: Erythromycin or clindamycin lotions or pads
                i.   Benzamycin or Benzaclin for patients with a mixture of
                         comodones and pustules
                ii.   Combination of benzoyl peroxide and drying agents
                         (Novacet, Sufacet)
        d.   Large open comedones (blackheads) should be expressed
3.   Moderate acne (or severe pustular acne) requires systemic antibiotics
        along with topical treatments
        a.   Doxycycline: 100 mg
        b.   Erythromycin: 1 gram in 2 to 3 divided doses
        c.   Minocycline: 50 to 100 mg twice a day
4.   Severe acne that does not respond to above should be treated with
        isotretinoin 0.5 to 1 mg/kg/day for 20 weeks (total 120 mg/kg);
        contraindicated in pregnancy
        a.   Requires baseline liver enzymes, cholesterol, and triglycerides
                prior to isotretinoin therapy
        b.   Females: Negative serum pregnancy test or two negative urine
                tests must be obtained during and 1 week prior to initiation of
                therapy; also effective contraception (suggest oral contraceptives
                such as Ortho Tri-Cyclen, Yasmin) must also be maintained during,
                and one month after therapy
        c.   Always obtain informed consent
        d.   For those with severe acne, unresponsive to conventional therapy,
                may also refer to dermatologist for dermabrasion, laser, or
                triamcinolone (Kenalog) injections

Fungal Infections

There are a variety of fungal infections that are distinguished by the causative species of fungi and the location they manifest.

1.   Fungal organisms Trichophyton (80%) or Microsporum cause the dermatophyte infections
2.   Pharmacologic management centers around anti-fungal therapy and prevention of transmission

Disorders

1.   Tinea capitus (scalp)
2.   Tinea corporis (body ringworm)
3.   Tinea cruris (jock itch)
4.   Tinea manuum and tinea pedis (athlete's foot)
5.   Tinea versicolor (hypo/hyperpigmentation macules on limbs)

Signs/Symptoms

1.   May be asymptomatic (e.g., tinea capitus)
2.   Some forms present with severe itching (tinea cruris and tinea pedis)
3.   Erythematous rings (tinea corporis)
4.   Solitary areas of hypopigmentation or hyperpigmentation (tinea versicolor)

Laboratory/Diagnostics

1.   "Spaghetti and meatballs" hyphae microscopically when treated with KOH

Management

1.   Tinea capitus: Selenium 2.5% shampoo twice weekly, griseofulvin 20 mg/kg/day × 6 weeks
2.   Tinea corporis: Use of topical antifungals is usually adequate (miconazole 2%, ketoconazole 2%)
3.   Tinea cruris: Any topical antifungal noted above; terbinafine cream curative in more than 80% of cases when used twice a day × 7 days; Griseofulvin for severe cases
4.   Tinea manuum and pedis: In macerated stage use, aluminum subacetate solution to soak for 20 minutes twice a day; apply topical antifungals as described in the dry, scaly stage; use oral therapy in severe cases
5.   Tinea versicolor: Selenium sulfide shampoo for 5 to 15 minutes daily × 7 days; 200 mg itraconazole (Sporonox) every day by mouth (alternative)

Varicella Zoster Virus (Chickenpox)

Acute, contagious disease caused by herpes virus, transmitted by direct contact with lesions or airborne

1.   Infected individuals are contagious for 48 hours before outbreak and until lesions have crusted over
2.   Most common in ages 5 to 10, in the late winter/early spring

Signs/Symptoms

1.   Erythematous macules
2.   Papules develop over macules
3.   Vesicles erupt
4.   Distributes primarily on trunk, scalp, face
5.   Intense pruritus
6.   Low grade fever
7.   Generalized lymphadenopathy

Laboratory/Diagnostics

1.   None, typically a clinical diagnosis

Management

1.   Prevention with vaccine
2.   Supportive treatment for pruritus
      a.   Calamine lotion
      b.   Antihistamine
      c.   Acetaminophen for fever
3.   Oral acyclovir 20 mg/kg four times a day; given in the first 24 hours, this can reduce the magnitude and/or duration of symptoms
4.   Intravenous (IV) acyclovir for immunocompromised patients

Molluscum Contagiosum

A benign, common viral skin infection; frequently these lesions disappear on their own in a few weeks to a few months and are not easily treated

1.   Diagnostic criteria include pruritus, the presence of very small, firm, pink to flesh-colored discrete papules, which become umbilicated papules with a cheesy core
2.   Children who are sexually active or abused can have grouped lesions in the genital area
3.   Children with eczema or immunosuppression can have severe infections

Signs/Symptoms

1.   Lesions present on the face, axillae, antecubital fossa, trunk, crural fascia, and extremities are most commonly noted
2.   Itching at the site of infection

Laboratory/Diagnostics

1.   Clinical presentation

2.   History of exposure to molluscum contagiosum

Management

Resolves spontaneously if left alone

1.   Mechanical removal of the central core prevents spread and autoinoculation
2.   Curettage, after anesthetizing the area with prilocaine 2.5% with lidocaine 2.5% cream (EMLA), is a useful treatment of a few lesions but should not be used on sensitive areas, since it may scar
3.   Pharmacological agents
    a.   Tretinoin 0.025% gel or 0.1% cream at bedtime (HS for "hour of sleep")
    b.   Salicylic acid daily at HS
    c.   Liquid nitrogen applied for 2 to 3 seconds
    d.   Tricholoracetic acid peel 25 to 50% applied by dropper to the center of lesion, followed by alcohol repeated every 2 weeks
    e.   Silver nitrate, iodine 7 to 9%, or phenol 1% applied for 2 to 3 seconds
    f.   Cantharidin 0.7% applied to individual lesions and covered with clear tape; blistering within 24 hours and possible clearing without scarring; should be avoided on facial lesions
4.   Prevent scratching and touching lesions to stop from spreading
5.   Spontaneous resolution may occur after 6 to 9 months in some immunocompetent patients
6.   If a patient has extensive lesions or the diagnosis is unclear, refer to dermatologist

Atopic Dermatitis (Eczema)

Chronic skin condition characterized by intense itching along a typical pattern of distribution with periods of remission and exacerbation

1.   Particularly sensitive to low humidity and often worsens in the winter when the air is dry
2.   Also helpful are a personal or family history of asthma, allergic rhinitis, atopic dermatitis, elevated serum IgE levels, and a tendency for skin infections

Signs/Symptoms

1.   Intense pruritus along face, neck, trunk, wrists, hands, antecubital and popliteal folds
2.   Dry scaly skin
    a.   Acute flare ups may show red patches that are red, shiny or thickened patches

   b.   Inflammed and/or scabbed lesions with diffuse erythema and
           scaling
   c.   Dry, leathery and lichenified skin

Laboratory/Diagnostics

1.   Scratch and intradermal tests often false positive
2.   RAST or skin tests may suggest dust mite allergy (food allergy uncommon)
3.   Serum IgE may be elevated; eosonphilia (elevated)

Management

1.   Dry skin management: Lotion immediately after bathing; must blot dry
        with towel first
2.   Topical steroids applied two to four times daily, rubbed in well; begin with
        hydrocortisone or other steroids (Fluocinonide cream 0.05%, Desonide,
        triamcinolone 0.1%); taper to avoid flare-ups
3.   Systemic steroids only in extremely severe cases: Prednisone 40 mg daily,
        taper down
4.   In acute weeping:
        a.   Use saline or aluminum subacetate solution
        b.   Colloidal oatmeal baths (e.g., Aveeno)

Allergic Contact Dermatitis

An acute or chronic dermatitis that results from direct skin contact with chemicals
or allergens

Signs/Symptoms

1.   Redness, pruritus, scabbing
2.   Tiny vesicles and weepy, encrusted lesions in acute phases
3.   Scaling, erythema and thickened skin (lichenfication) in chronic phase
4.   Location will suggest cause
5.   Affected areas hot and swollen
6.   History of exposure to the offending agent

Laboratory/Diagnostics

1.   None indicated

Management

1.   Depends on severity; compresses locally, avoid scrub with soap and water
2.   High potency topical steroids locally
3.   If severe and systemic: Prednisone starting at 60 mg daily and tapering
        over 14 days

161

Irritant (Diaper) Dermatitis

Common skin irritation of the genital-perianal region

1.　Most common type of diaper rash, typically due to exposure to chemical irritants and prolonged contact with urine and/or feces
2.　Occurs at some time in 95% of infants; peaks at 9 to 12 months

Signs/Symptoms

1.　Fiery red rash
2.　Papules, vesicles, crusts, ulcerations
3.　Infant may be irritable

Laboratory/Diagnostics

1.　None indicated

Management

1.　In mild cases, barrier emollients
2.　When erythema/papules present, 1% hydrocortisone
3.　Use Burrow's compresses for severe erythema and vesicles
4.　Secondary bacterial infection may need topical antibiotics
5.　Secondary fungus may need topical antifungal
6.　Educate parents about preventive measures
7.　Avoid plastic pants
8.　Allow diaper area to air several times daily

Psoriasis

A common benign hyperproliferative inflammatory skin disorder (acute or chronic) based on genetic predisposition (affecting approximately 35% of the population)

1.　The epidermal turnover time is reduced from 14 days to 2 days
2.　Normal maturation of the skin cells cannot take place, and keratinization is faulty
3.　The epidermis is thickened, and immature nucleated cells are seen on the horny layer
4.　May be immunologically mediated

Signs/Symptoms

1.　Often asymptomatic; itching may occur
2.　Lesions are red, sharply defined plaques with silvery scales
3.　Scalp, elbows, knees, palms, soles, and nails are common sites
4.　Fine pitting of the nails is strongly suggestive of psoriasis, as is separation of the nail plate from the bed
5.　Pink or red line in the intergluteal fold

6.   Auspitz sign: Droplets of blood when scales are removed

Laboratory/Diagnostics

1.   None indicated

Management

1.   Topicals for the scalp
      a.   Tar/salicylic acid shampoo
      b.   Medium potency topical steroid oil
2.   Topicals for the skin
      a.   Topical steroids twice a day × 2 to 3 weeks (not 1 week); resume with calciportriene (Dovonex), a synthetic Vitamin B3 derivative
      b.   Bethamethasone dipropionate 0.05% (Diprolene AF)
      c.   Triamcinolone acetonide 0.5% (Aristrocort)
3.   UVB light and coal tar exposure if more than 30% of the body surface is involved
4.   Moisturizers

Pityriasis Rosea

A mild, acute inflammatory disorder; usually self-limiting, lasting 3 to 8 weeks

1.   If the cause is unknown, the current theory is that it is viral in origin
2.   More common in the spring and fall seasons, and patients frequently report a recent upper respiratory infection (URI)
3.   More common in females than males

Signs/Symptoms

1.   May be asymptomatic
2.   Initial lesion (2 to 10 cm) known as "herald patch"
      a.   Usually macular, oval, and fawn-colored with a crinkled appearance and collarette scale
3.   Puritic rash in a Christmas tree pattern (usually mild) may be found on the trunk and proximal extremities within 1 to 2 weeks

Laboratory/Diagnostics

1.   Serologic test for syphilis should be performed
      a.   If the rash does not itch
      b.   If the palmar and plantar surfaces or mucous membranes are involved
      c.   If a few typically perfect lesions are not present

Management

1.   None usually required
2.   If pruritic:

      a.   Atarax

      b.   Oral antihistamines [e.g., loratadine (Claritan), fexofenadine (Allegra), cartirizine (Zyrtec)]

      c.   Topical antipruritic (Sarna lotion, Prax lotion, itch-Xgel, Cetaphil with menthol 0.25% and phenol 0.25%)

      d.   Cool compresses, baths (with or without colloidal oatmeal)

      e.   Topical steroids (medium strength): Triamcinolone 0.1%

3.   Daily sunlight exposure will hasten healing; most effectively ultraviolet B daily × 1 week

4.   Oral erythromycin (2 week course) is effective in the majority of patients

Impetigo

A bacterial infection of the skin typically caused by gram positive strep or staph (Staph aureus) organisms

1.   Involves the face predominately but can occur anywhere on the body

2.   Occurs most often in the summer

3.   Highly contagious and autoinoculable

Signs/Symptoms

1.   Signs of inflammation

2.   Pain, swelling, warmth

3.   Regional lymphandenopathy

4.   Classic honey-crusting lesions

Laboratory/Diagnostics

1.   None indicated, clinical diagnosis

2.   Culture would confirm causative organism if desired

      a.   Systemic infection

      b.   Fever, chills

      c.   Malaise

      d.   Anorexia

      e.   Bullous impetigo (variant)

Management

1.   Systemic treatment should be directed at the offending organism

2.   Use atopical antimicrobials for minor infections (Bacitracin, Bactroban, etc.)

3.   Based on organism: Use the oral beta lactamase resistant antibiotics when oral route preferred

      a.   Staphylococcus aureas

          i.   Anti-staphyloccal antibiotics: Dicloxacillan, Cephalexin, Erythromycin, Clindamycin

      b.   Streptococcus

      i.   Topical mupirocin or fusidic acid are very effective for the streptococcal lesion, with or without staphyloccal overgrowth

      ii.   If nephritogenic strain of streptococcus is suspected, systemic antibiotic therapy with PCN is indicated

  c.   Severe cellulitis: IV antibiotics (nafcillin, vancomycin, doxycycline)

4. Certain infections may require surgical excision of the affected area
5. Abstain from school and other community events for 48 hours
6. Apply Burrow's solution to clean lesions

Scabies

Highly contagious skin infestation caused by a parasitic mite that burrows into stratum corneum

1. Incubation of 4 to 6 weeks
2. Spread via direct or indirect contact with personal items

Signs/Symptoms

1. Intense itching
2. Irritability in infants
3. Linear curved burrows
4. Infants: Red-brown vesiculopapular lesions on head, neck, palms, or soles
5. Older children: Red papules on skin folds, umbilicus, or abdomen
6. May see regional adenopathy

Laboratory/Diagnostics

1. Skin scrapings show mites, ova, and/or feces
2. None typically necessary

Management

1. Permethrin (Nix) 5% rinse for 8 to 14 hours, repeat in 1 week, or:
2. Lindane lotion (Kwell): Apply once and wash off in 8 to 12 hours; do not retreat
3. Rash may persist for 1 week
4. Wash all washable items
5. Store non washable items for 1 week
6. Antihistamines for pruritus

Lyme Disease

A spirochetal disease, the most common vector-borne disease in the United States

1. Most cases occur in the Northeast, Upper Midwest, and Pacific Coast

2.   Mice and deer ticks are the major animal reservoirs, but birds may also be a source

Etiology/Incidence

1.   Borrelia burgdorferi (Spirochete)
2.   Ticks must feed more than 24 to 36 hours to transmit infecting organism
3.   Congenital infection has been documented but is questionable

Signs/Symptoms

Stage 1

1.   Erythema migrans: A flat or slightly raised red lesion that expands over several days but has central clearing; commonly appears in areas of tight clothing
2.   50% of patients have flu-like symptoms

Stage 2

1.   Headache, stiff joints
2.   Migratory pains
3.   Some patients may have cardiac symptoms (dysrhythmias, heart block)
4.   Asceptic meningitis
5.   Bell's palsy
6.   Peripheral neuropathy

Stage 3

1.   Joint and periarticular pain
2.   Subacute encephalopathy
3.   Acrodermatitis chronicum atrophicans: Bluish red discoloration of the distal extremity with edema

Laboratory/Diagnostics

1.   Detection of antibody to B. burgdorferi via ELISA screening
2.   Western blot assay is confirmatory
3.   B. burgdorferi may be cultured from skin aspirate
4.   Elevated ESR
5.   Diagnostic criteria
    a.   Exposure to tick habitat within the last 30 days with:
        i.   Erythema migrans
            OR
        ii.   One late manifestation
            AND
    b.   Laboratory confirmation

Management

1. Infection confined to the skin
   a. Under age 9: PCN VK or Amoxicillin
   b. Over age 9: Amoxicillin or Doxycycline
2. Referral for stage 2 or 3 disease

Rubella

An acute, contagious viral disease caused by an RNA virus known for its teratogenicity

Signs/Symptoms

1. History of inadequate immunization
2. Fine erythematous maculopapular rash begins on face, spreads to extremities and trunk; gone within 72 hours
3. Associated malaise
4. Joint pain
5. Postauricular and suboccipital lymphadenopathy

Laboratory/Diagnostics

1. A variety of assays available

Management

1. Supportive: Fever with acetaminophen
2. Educate regarding danger to pregnant women

Erythema Infectiosum (Fifth Disease)

A contagious exanthematous disease caused by human parvovirus B19

1. Occurs most often in the spring in children aged 5 to 14
2. Transmitted via respiratory droplets and infected blood
3. Incubates 4 to 14 days

Signs/Symptoms

1. Sudden onset "slapped cheek" appearance: Lacy reticular exanthema
2. Spreads to upper arms, legs, trunks, and dorsum of the hands/feet
3. Rash can last up to 40 days; average of 1.5 weeks
4. Can cause aplastic crisis

Laboratory/Diagnostics

1. Parvovirus B19 IgM, IgG

Management

1.   None needed
2.   Patient education: Intrauterine infection can produce fetal anemia
3.   Immunoglobulin to exposed pregnant women

Coxsackie Virus (Hand-Foot-And-Mouth-Disease)

A highly contagious vial illness resulting in ulceration and inflammation of the soft palate (herpangina) and papulovesicular exanthem on the hands and feet

1.   Affects children over 10 years of age
2.   Resolves spontaneously in less than a week
3.   There is evidence of a relationship between coxsackie and diabetes mellitus

Signs/Symptoms

1.   Fever
2.   Malaise
3.   Vomiting
4.   Drooling
5.   Papulovesicular rash as described

Laboratory/Diagnostics

1.   None indicated

Management

1.   Acetaminophen
2.   Topical applications for comfort

Sample Questions

1. A mother brings her newly-adopted daughter from Russia into the clinic after noticing a rash all over her body. Upon examination, you notice that the rash consists of erythematous macules concentrated on the face, scalp, and trunk. Some of the papules and erupted vesicles are also noted. The patient also has a low grade fever and has been scratching during the entire exam. Which of the following dermatologic conditions is most likely?

   a. Varicella zoster
   b. Tinea corporis
   c. Atopic dermatitis
   d. Pityriasis rosea

2. Impetigo is a bacterial infection of the skin that involves predominately the face but can occur anywhere on the body. The organisms most responsible are:

   a. Haemophilus influenza and Escherichia
   b. Streptococcus pneumoniae or Neisseria
   c. Gram positive Streptococcus or Staph aureus
   d. Streptococcus pneumoniae and Escherichia

3. A toddler presents to the clinic with a fine erythematous maculopapular rash that started on the face one day ago but has now spread to the extremities and trunk. What is the most likely dermatologic condition?

   a. Rubella
   b. Pityriasis Rosea
   c. Scabies
   d. Impetigo

Answers

1. Correct Answer: A
Atopic dermatitis, varicella zoster, and pityriasis rosea all include pruitis. There is often a low grade fever with varicella zoster but not the other 2. Atopic dermatitis features dry scaly, skin. Varicella zoster has macules that form papules over them along with vesicles that erupt and then crust over.

2. Correct Answer: C
Bacterial infections of the skin are typically caused by gram positive *Streptococcus* or staph (*Staph aureus*) organisms. These occur most often in the summer, are highly contagious, and are autoinoculable.

3. Correct Answer: A
Scabies is a red-brown vesiculopapular lesion on the head, neck, palms, and soles. Impetigo is a honey colored crusted lesions. Pityriasis rosea has herald patches and a Christmas tree-pattern appearance. Rubella has the rash described that spreads and resolves within 72 hours.

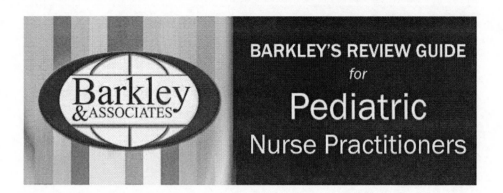

Eye, Ear, Nose, and Throat Issues and Disorders

Hordeolum (Stye)

A common staphylococcal abscess on the upper or lower eyelid

1. External hordeolum is on the lid margin (points toward the eyelid skin surface); most common presentation
2. Internal hordeolum is a sebacceous gland abscess that points toward the conjunctival surface

Causes/Incidence

1. Staphylococcus
2. Extremely common

Differential Diagnosis

1. Conjunctivitis
2. Chalazion
3. Blepharitis
4. Dacrocystitis

Signs/Symptoms

1. Abrupt onset
2. Localized pain (acutely tender) and edema
3. Pain proportional to the amount of edema

Management

1. Warm compresses
2. Topical bacitracin or erythromycin ophthalmic ointment may be considered
3. Refer to ophthalmologist for possible incision and drainage (I&D) if there is no resolution within 48 hours

Chalazion

A granulomatous (beady nodule) on the eyelid; infection or retention cyst of the meibomian gland

Note: A chalazion is a hard, non-tender cyst; it differs from styes (hordeolums) in that chalazians are usually painless.

Signs/Symptoms

1. Asymptomatic
2. Red conjunctiva
3. Itching
4. Visual distortion if the cyst is large enough to impress cornea; may cause astigmatism (blurred vision) due to pressure on the cornea
5. Eyelid swelling
6. Light sensitivity
7. Increased tearing

Management

1. Warm compresses
2. Referral for surgical removal

Conjunctivitis

The most common eye disorder; an inflammation/infection of the conjunctiva ("pink eye") resulting from a variety of causes including allergies, chemical irritation, or infection (bacterial, viral, gonococcal/chlamydial)

Signs/Symptoms

1. Inflammation, redness, irritation
2. Itching, burning
3. Increased tears
4. Blurred vision possible
5. Eyelid swelling
6. Foreign body sensation
7. Eyelids may be crusty and sticky with mucopurulent discharge

Laboratory / Diagnostics

1. Gram stain and culture when indicated (e.g., if gonococcal is suspected)

Management

Type	Discharge	Treatment Considerations
Chemical		1. Self-limiting 2. No treatment required
Bacterial	Purulent	1. Erythromycin 0.5% ophthalmic ointment 2. Tetracycline 1% 3. Polymyxin B ophthalmic solution or ointment
Bacterial:	Copious, Purulent	
1. Gonococcal (Ophthalmic emergency)		IV Pen G or ceftriaxone 250 mg IM
2. Chlamydia		Erythromycin ophthalmic ointment Oral: Tetracycline*, erythromycin, clarithromycin*, azithromycin, doxycycline*
Allergic	Stringy; increased tearing	1. Oral antihistamines 2. Refer to allergist/ophthalmologist 3. May need steroids
Viral 1. Adenovirus	Watery	Symptomatic care 1. *Mild*: Saline gtts/artificial tears (refrigerated, cool is best) 2. *Moderate*: Decongestants/antihistamines, mast cell stabilizers, NSAIDS
2. Herpetic	Bright red and irritated	Refer to Ophthalmologist
* Note: Safe in pregnancy		

1. To decrease bacterial resistance, avoid chronic use or empiric broad-spectrum antibiotics especially for self-limiting types (chemical, adenovirus, and allergic)
2. Avoid steroids which tend to activate or accelerate unrecognized herpes simplex virus infections; chronic use may raise intraocular pressure and cause cataracts later in life

Cataracts

An abnormal, uniform, progressive opacity of the eye seen in children with co-morbid syndromes (e.g., Down syndrome, diabetes mellitus, Marfan's syndrome and atopic dermatitis)

Causes/Incidence

1. Congenital
2. Prolonged steroid use
3. Infection
4. Injury
5. Radiation

Signs/Symptoms

1. Painless
2. Decreased visual acuity
3. Clouded, blurred, dim vision
4. White fundus reflex
5. Poor visual fixation
6. Photophobia

Laboratory/Diagnostics

1. None indicated

Management

1. Refer for surgical removal

Retinoblastoma

A congenital malignant intraocular tumor that can be hereditary or acquired; occurs in 1:10,000 children

1. Usually diagnosed before age 5
2. Peak incidence is around 18 months

Signs/Symptoms

1. Squinting
2. Eyes turn inward or outward
3. Painful red eye
4. Leukocoria (yellow-white papillary reflex)
5. Hyphema
6. Stabismus
7. Creamy pink mass on fundoscopic exam

<u>**Diagnostic Studies**</u>

1.   CT or MRI of the orbits: Evaluate extent of optic nerve or bony involvement

<u>**Management**</u>

1.   Refer for surgical resection or enucleating
2.   Radiation
3.   Chemotherapy

Strabismus

1.   Ocular misalignment as a result of uncoordinated ocular muscles
2.   If acquired after 6 months of age, it is usually related to an underlying problem

<u>**Signs/Symptoms**</u>

1.   Squinting
2.   Decreased visual acuity
3.   Head tilt
4.   Face turning
5.   Esotropia: Eyes deviate inward
6.   Exotropia: Eyes deviate outward
7.   Hypertropia: Eyes deviate upward
8.   Hypotropia: Eyes deviate downward
9.   Hirschberg papillary light reflex is unequal

<u>**Management**</u>

1.   Refer to ophthalmology:
    a.   If fixed or continuous at 6 months of age or more
    b.   Immediately for hypertropia (an upward deviation of the eye) and hypotropia (a disorder in which two eyes do not line up in the same direction)
    c.   Signs of underlying cause present
2.   Specialist plan for treatment
    a.   Patching
    b.   Orthoptic exercises
    c.   Surgical correction

Otitis Externa (Swimmer's ear)

Inflammation of the external auditory meatus

<u>**Causes/Incidence**</u>

1.   Infection
    a.   Bacterial (usually gram-negative)

      b.   Fungal
      c.   Viral

2. Recent history of water exposure
3. History of mechanical trauma, foreign body, or excess cerumen may be present

Signs/Symptoms

1. Otalgia
2. Pruritus
3. Purulent discharge

Physical Exam Findings

1. Erythema of the ear canal
2. Edema of the ear canal
3. Purulent exudate (sometimes with odor)
4. Pain upon manipulation of auricle
5. Lateral surface of tympanic membrane may be erythematous
6. Tympanic membrane: Normal

Laboratory/Diagnostics

1. Pneumatic otoscopy should demonstrate mobility

Management

1. Remove purulent debris
2. Protect from moisture or injury
3. Topical ear medications:
      a.   Bacterial:
            i.   Acetic acid with or without hydrocortisone
            ii.   Corticosporin (Neomycin, polymyxin B, HC)
            iii.   Ciprofloxacin or Ofloxacin for severe cases
      b.   Fungal:
            i.   Antifungal drops (e.g., clotrimazole 1% solution)

Acute Otitis Media (AOM)

Bacterial infection of the mucosally lined air-containing spaces of temporal bone

Causes/Incidence

Bacterial:
      a.   *Streptococcus pneumoniae* (30%)
      b.   *Haemophilus influenzae* (20%)
Viral:
      a.   RSV
      b.   *Influenzae*

c.   *M. pneumoniae*
Fungal: Rare

Signs/Symptoms

1.   Decreased hearing
2.   Otalgia
3.   Fever
4.   Aural pressure
5.   Vertigo
6.   Nausea/vomiting

Physical Exam Findings

1.   Tympanic membrane
      a.   Erythematous
      b.   Edematous
2.   Purulent exudate
3.   Tympanic membrane rarely bulges

Laboratory/Diagnostics

1.   Usually a clinical diagnosis
2.   Impaired mobility of tympanic membrane with pneumatic otoscopy
3.   Tympanometry
4.   Tympanocentesis and culture only in special circumstances

Management

1.   Pain management: Acetaminophen or ibuprofen; benzocaine otic drops
      for children > 5 years of age
2.   Observation period for healthy children: "Watchful waiting" for 48 to 72
      hours
3.   Medications:
      a.   Amoxicillin 80 to 90mg/kg/day, twice daily orally × 10 days (if > 6
            years of age and mild to moderate disease is apparent: Use 5 to
            7 day course)
      b.   If the child is allergic, may use cefdinir (Omnicef), cefpodoxime
            (Vantin), or cefuroxime (Ceftin/Zinacef)

Serous Otitis Media/Otis Media with Effusion (OME)

The presence of fluid in the middle ears without the signs or symptoms of AOM;
also known as chronic otitis media with effusion

Causes/Incidence

1.   Blocked eustachian tubes; inability to equalize pressure
2.   Allergy, barotrauma influence

<u>**Signs/Symptoms**</u>

1.   Hearing loss
2.   Popping sensation when pressure altered
3.   Fullness in the ear

<u>**Physical Exam Findings**</u>

1.   Air bubbles behind the tympanic membrane
2.   Decreased membrane mobility
3.   Weber and Rinne tests suggestive of conductive hearing loss

<u>**Laboratory/Diagnostics**</u>

1.   Decreased hearing via audiometry

<u>**Management**</u>

1.   Watchful monitoring: 3 months
2.   Antibiotic therapy: No long-term efficacy
3.   Antihistamines/decongestants: Ineffective
4.   Re-evaluate in 3 to 6 months

Hearing Loss

Any degree of impairment in the ability to apprehend sound

1.   May be conductive or sensorineural

<u>**Conduction Causes**</u>

Decreased ability to conduct sound from external to inner ear
1.   Cerumen impaction/foreign body (most treatable)
2.   Hematoma
3.   Otitis media
4.   Perforated tympanic membrane
5.   Otosclerosis
6.   Cholesteatoma

<u>**Sensorineural Loss**</u>

Impaired transmission of sound through the nervous system

<u>**Causes**</u>

1.   Acoustic neuroma
2.   Syphilis
3.   Central nervous system disease
4.   Medication toxicity

<u>Signs/Symptoms</u>

1.   Understanding Weber and Rinne Tests
2.   Normal Findings:
        a.   Weber test: Sound should be heard equally in both ears and not
                lateralize
        b.   Rinne test: Air conduction (AC) > bone conduction (BC)
3.   Findings with hearing loss
        a.   Conductive hearing loss:
                i.   Weber test: Sound lateralizes to the affected ear
                ii.   Rinne test: Abnormal in affected ear (i.e., AC < BC)
        b.   Sensorineural hearing loss:
                i.   Weber test: Sound lateralizes to the unaffected ear
                ii.   Rinne test: Normal in the affected ear

<u>Laboratory/Diagnostics</u>

1.   Otoscopic exam: Inspect canal and tympanic membrane
2.   General neurological exam
3.   Audiometric testing
4.   CT scan if a neurologic condition is suspected
5.   Serum blood tests as needed

<u>Management</u>

1.   Remove foreign body/cerumen
2.   Refer for audiogram
3.   Refer for further evaluation/hearing aid

Common Cold

Viral rhinitis, a self-limiting upper respiratory tract infection

<u>Causes/Incidence</u>

1.   Rhinoviruses, adenoviruses
2.   Incidence decreases with age

<u>Signs/Symptoms</u>

1.   Headache
2.   Watery rhinorrhea
3.   Sneezing
4.   Cough
5.   Sore throat
6.   Malaise

<u>Differential Diagnosis</u>

1.   Sinusitis

2. Influenza
3. Allergic rhinitis
4. Strep throat

Physical Findings

1. Edematous nasal mucosa
2. Erythematous nasal mucosa
3. Erythematous pharynx
4. Watery eyes
5. Lungs clear to auscultation

Laboratory/Diagnostics

1. None
2. Throat culture if strep infection suspected

Management

1. Rest and hydration
2. Over the counter analgesics
3. Cough management
4. Nasal saline drops
5. No OTC cold preparations (e.g., decongestants, antihistamines, antitussives, expectorants)

Pharyngitis/Tonsillitis

Inflammation of the pharynx or tonsils

Causes/Incidence

1. Viruses (RSV, influenza A; B, Epstein Barr virus)
2. Group A B-hemolytic streptococci
3. *Neisseria gonorrhoeae*
4. Mycoplasma
5. *Chlamydia trachomatis*
6. Corynebacterium sp.

Signs/Symptoms

1. Erythematous pharynx
2. Dysphagia; cough
3. Malaise
4. Rhinorrhea (viral)
5. Fever (more pronounced in bacterial infections)
6. Anterior cervical adenopathy (bacterial)
7. Painful throat
8. Exudate

Centor criteria:

Clinical features most suggestive of group A beta-hemolytic streptococci (GABHS) include **FLEA**:

1. **F**ever > 98°F
2. **L**ack of cough
3. Pharyngotonsillar **E**xudate
4. **A**nterior cervical adenopothy

Differential Diagnosis

1. Epiglottitis
2. Abscess

Physical Exam Findings

1. Erythematous pharynx
2. Exudate (bacterial)
3. Anterior cervical adenopathy (bacterial)

Laboratory/Diagnostics

1. Throat culture
2. White blood cell (WBC) count elevated in bacterial infection

Management

1. Fluids/hydration
2. Warm salt water gargles
3. Antipyretics (acetaminophen or ibuprofen)
4. Medications:
   a. Antibiotics for streptococcal infection
      i. Penicillin VK 250 mg orally three times daily × 10 days
      ii. If allergic to PCN> Erythromycin 250 mg four times daily × 10 days
   b. Gonococcal management:
      i. Ceftriaxone 125 mg intramuscular (IM) once
      ii. Ofloxacin 400 mg orally once
      iii. Cefixime 400 mg orally once
      iv. Treat for Chlamydia
5. Refer as appropriate

Epiglottitis

Sudden, severe swelling of the epiglottis that occurs as a result of bacterial infection; can produce respiratory compromise in a matter of hours

1. Common pathogens include Streptococci, Pneumococci, and H. influenzae

2.   Peak incidence occurs between ages 6 and 10

Signs/Symptoms

1.   Sudden onset high fever
2.   Drooling
3.   Choking sensation
4.   Restless, fearful
5.   Hyperextension of the neck
6.   Rapidly progressive signs of respiratory distress

Laboratory/Diagnostics

1.   Blood and tracheal cultures for causative organism
2.   "Thumb sign," a thumb-shaped patch, appearing on a radiograph of the neck

Management

1.   Immediate hospitalization
2.   Do not perform a pharyngeal exam
3.   Keep child calm
4.   Intubation capabilities as soon as possible
5.   IV third generation cephalosporin until pathogen identified

Croup

Parainfluenza viral infection of the larynx

1.   Severity can range from mild to quite severe
2.   Peak incidence is from 3 months to 6 years of age
3.   Affects males more often than females
4.   Most common in fall and winter

Signs/Symptoms

1.   Recent symptoms of an upper respiratory infect (URI)
2.   Bark-like cough
3.   Low grade fever
4.   Vital signs consistent with infection
5.   Dyspnea
6.   Stridor if severe
7.   Lungs typically clear

Laboratory/Diagnostics

1.   Pulse oximtery: Shows hypoxic in severe forms
2.   Appearance of a "steeple"-shaped narrowing of the trachea on a frontal radiograph of the neck

Management

1.	Mild disease: Outpatient supportive care
2.	Moderate disease: Hospitalize for respiratory support; IV fluids
3.	May require nebulized racemic epinephrine
4.	Short course of corticosteroids

Epiglottitis vs. Croup

Epiglottitis	Croup
Bacterial infection	Viral infection, bacteria rare
Supraglottic structure	Larynx
6 to 10 years of age	3 months to 6 years of age
High fever, drooling	Low fever, "barky cough"
X-ray: thumb sign	X-ray: steeple sign

Infectious Mononucleosis

An acute infectious disease due to the Epstein-Barr virus, usually occurring over the age of 10

1.	Mode of transmission is saliva
2.	Incubation period: One to 2 months
3.	Usually self-limited, but malaise and fatigue may last months

Signs/Symptoms

1.	Fever
2.	Pharyngitis (most severe)
3.	Malaise, anorexia, myalgia

Physical Exam Findings

1.	Cervical adenopathy or lymphadenopathy: Posterior cervical lymphadenopathy may be present
2.	White exudate on tonsils may be present
3.	Splenomegaly
4.	Maculopapular or petechial rash

Laboratory/Diagnostics

1.	Lymphocytic leukocytosis; neutropenia
2.	Positive heterophil and monospot
3.	Early rise in Immunoglobulin M (IgM)

4.   Permanent rise in Immunoglobulin G (IgG)

Management

1.   Supportive (e.g., non-steroidals, warm saline gargles)
2.   Corticosteroids when enlarged lymph tissue threatens airway obstruction
3.   Avoidance of contact sports (3 weeks to several months) to avoid splenic rupture (even without clinically detectable splenomegaly)

Sinusitis (Rhinosinusitis)

Occurs when an undrained collection of pus accumulates in 1 or more of the paranasal sinuses

1.   Can also result from dental infection; teeth that are tender should be checked for abscess
2.   Diseases that swell the nasal membrane, such as viral or allergic rhinitis, are usually the cause; 5 to 10% of URIs in children develop into sinusitis
3.   The maxillary and ethmoid sinuses are the most commonly affected
4.   Typical pathogens are the same as those of acute otitis media: *S. pneumoniae, H. influenzae,* and *M. catarrhalis*

Signs/Symptoms

1.   Pain and pressure over the cheek
2.   Headache
3.   Discolored nasal discharge; halitosis
4.   Post nasal drip and cough (usually during the day and may be worse at night)
5.   Dull, throbbing pain worsening when head is dependent

Laboratory/Diagnostics

1.   Diagnosis is often made on clinical presentation
2.   Radiological studies are not needed in uncomplicated presentations
   a.   Typical x-ray series (Caldwell, Waters, lateral and submentovertical) are not useful except for maxillary sinuses; will show opacification without bone destruction
   b.   CT scan preferred over standard x-rays because it is more sensitive and no more expensive; only for more complicated sinusitis
   c.   May culture purulent nasal discharge

Management

1.   Uncomplicated with mild symptoms treat as outpatient
   a.   Antibiotic therapy
      i.   Amoxicillin or erythromycin for 14 days; should see noticeable improvement in 3 to 4 days

        ii.   For unresponsive, chronic sinusitis or for patients in an area of high prevalence of beta-lactamase-producing *H. influenzae*, use amoxicillin-clavulanate, cefuroxime axetil or a newer macrolide

   b.   Decongestants, antihistamines are not useful in acute sinusitis; maybe in chronic sinusitis

   c.   Pain managed with acetaminophen or ibuprofen

   d.   Nighttime humidification to reduce mucosal drying

   e.   Increase fluids for hydration

2.   Chronic or recurrent sinusitis: Refer to otolaryngologist

Sample Questions

1. A 14-year-old presents with a hard non-tender cyst on the eyelid with no other signs or symptoms. Which of the following is the most likely diagnosis?

    a. Hordeolum
    b. Conjunctivitis
    c. Chalazion
    d. Dacryocystitis

2. A 7-year-old who is on the swim team comes in complaining of purulent discharge and pain in the left ear. Upon examination, you notice that the child appears to be in pain upon manipulation of the auricle, but the tympanic membrane appears normal and shows evidence of mobility. What is the most likely diagnosis?

    a. Acute otitis media
    b. Serous otitis media
    c. Otitis externa
    d. Mastoiditis

3. A 15-year-old male comes into the clinic complaining of general malaise and fatigue that have lasted for a few weeks without resolution. He has also had a fever and sore throat. All of the following exam findings would support the diagnosis of infectious mononucleosis, except:

    a. Diffuse cervical lymphadenopathy
    b. Maculopapular rash
    c. White exudate on tonsils
    d. Hepatomegaly

Answers

1. Correct Answer: C

Hordeolum and dacrocystitis are painful. Dactrocystitis is also red and inflamed. Conjunctivitis affects the conjunctiva and not the eyelid.

2. Correct Answer: C

Serous otitits media and acute otitis media would have decreased mobility of the membrane. Mastoiditis would have erythema and swelling noted over the mastoid region behind the ear. Otitis externa is also known as swimmer's ear and has the signs and symptoms listed.

3. Correct Answer: D

Splenomegaly, not hepatomegaly, is found in infectious mononucleosis. All other listed exam findings are indicative of infectious mononucleosis.

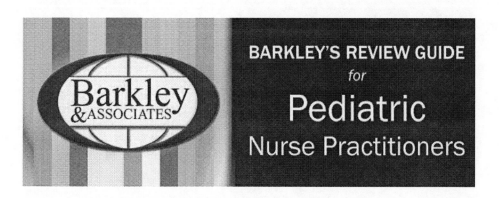

Respiratory Issues and Disorders

Pulmonary Functions Tests

Forced vital capacity (FVC)	Volume of gas forcefully expelled from the lungs after maximal inspiration
Forced expiratory volume (FEV1)	Volume of gas expelled in the first second of the FVC maneuver
FEV 25 to 75%	Maximal mid-expiratory airflow rate
Peak expiratory flow rate (PEFR)	Maximal airflow rate achieved in FVC maneuver
Total lung capacity (TLC)	Volume of gas in lungs after maximal inspiration
Functional residual capacity (FRC)	Functional residual capacity
Residual volume (RV)	Volume of gas remaining in lungs after maximal expiration
Obstructive Disease	1. Characterized by reduced airflow rates; lung volumes within normal range or larger 2. Typical of a child having trouble exhaling (air trapping) which results in decreased rates and FEV1 (e.g., asthma, chronic bronchitis, emphysema)
Restrictive Disease	1. Characterized by reduced volumes and expiratory flow rates 2. Typical of a child that has trouble inhaling air, thus affecting the volume (e.g., Pneumonia)

Bronchiolitis

A disease of the lower respiratory tract that causes inflammation leading to obstruction of the small respiratory airways

1.   Typically noted among children less than 3 years of age, this is a viral illness with respiratory syncytial virus (RSV) responsible for more than 50% of cases
2.   Parainfluenza virus (type 3), mycoplasma, or adenoviruses are usually the cause of the remaining 50% of cases.

Signs/Symptoms

1.   Upper respiratory infection (URI) symptoms lasting for several days
2.   Moderate fever to 102°F (38.9°C)
3.   Decrease in appetite
4.   Gradual development of respiratory distress (nasal flaring, grunting, cyanosis, prolonged expiration)
5.   Tachypnea (60 to 80/min)
6.   Non-productive cough
7.   Paroxysmal wheezing
8.   Palpable liver and spleen (pushed down due to hyperinflated lungs)
9.   Severe distress includes:
      a.   Progressive stridor
      b.   Stridor at rest
      c.   Increasing respiratory rate
      d.   Restlessness
      e.   Hypoxia
      f.   Rising PCO2 (per blood gas evaluation)
      g.   Pallor
      h.   Cyanosis
      i.   Depressed sensorium

Laboratory/Diagnostics

1.   Chest x-ray with hyperinflated lungs and increased A-P diameter; may have scattered areas of consolidation or inflammation of the alveoli
2.   Immunofluorescence analysis of nasal washing may be positive for RSV

Management

1.   Infants younger than 2 months and older infants with severe respiratory distress should be hospitalized
2.   Infants with mild distress can be treated as outpatients
      a.   Hydration
      b.   Antipyretics
      c.   Saline nasal drops
      d.   Give smaller, more frequent feedings, monitoring respiratory rate and guard against vomiting
3.   Prevention of RSV in high-risk infants with Synagis at 15 mg/kg intramuscularly every month during RSV season; the criteria for those who should receive palivizumab (Synagis) include:

a.   Less than 2 years of age with chronic lung disease treated within 6 months of RSV season

b.   Premature infant (< than 32 weeks gestation) during the first year of life

c.   Infants between 32 to 35 weeks gestation may be treated if the following risk factors are present:

    i.   Day care attendance
    ii.   School-aged siblings
    iii.   Exposure to environmental pollution
    iv.   Abnormal airways
    v.   Severe neuromuscular problems

Asthma

A disease characterized by an increased responsiveness of the trachea and bronchi to various stimuli, and manifested by widespread narrowing of the airways that changes in severity either spontaneously or as a result of treatment

Pathophysiology

1. Hypertrophy of smooth muscle
2. Mucosal edema and hyperemia
3. Thickening of epithelial basement membrane
4. Hypertrophy of mucus glands
5. Acute inflammation and plugging of airways by thick, viscid mucus
6. Can be triggered by allergens, exercise, drugs, or cardiac conditions

Causes

Most common allergens are encountered indoors

1.   Dust mites
2.   Pets (cat, dog)
3.   Cockroaches
4.   Indoor molds
5.   Exercise
6.   Airway irritants
    a.   Cigarettes
    b.   Air pollution (including ozone)
    c.   Wood smoke
    d.   Perfumes
    e.   Aerosol sprays
    f.   Paints or sealants
    g.   Cleaning agents
7.   Cold air
8.   Medications (e.g., aspirin)
9.   Food (e.g., yellow dye)

10.   Stress
11.   Infections
     a.   Colds
     b.   Sinus infections
     c.   Bronchitis

Signs/Symptoms

1.   Respiratory distress at rest
2.   Difficulty speaking in sentences
3.   Diaphoresis
4.   Use of accessory muscles
5.   Pulsus paradoxus > 12 mm Hg
6.   Hyperresonance
7.   Cough
8.   Chest tightness

Ominous signs include:
1.   Fatigue
2.   Absent breath sounds
3.   Pulsus paradoxus
4.   Inability to maintain recumbency
5.   Cyanosis

Laboratory/Diagnostics

1.   Slight white blood cell elevation with eosinophilia
2.   Pulmonary function tests (PFTs) reveal abnormalities typical of obstructive dysfunction
3.   Hospitalization is recommended if:
     a.   The initial Forced Expiratory Volume in the first second (FEV1) is more than 30% predicted or does not increase to at least 40% predicted after 1 hour of vigorous therapy
     b.   The peak flow is less than 60 liters/minute initially or does not improve to more than 50% predicted after 1 hour of treatment
4.   Will generally see improvement in Forced Vital Capacity (FVC) or FEV1 of 15% or FEV 25 to75 of 25% after inhaled bronchodilator
5.   A chest x-ray is unnecessary unless used to rule out other conditions; may show hyperinflation

Classification of Severity

Classification	Days with Symptoms	Night With Symptoms	PEV or FEV1 ↑	PEF Variability
Severe Persistent	Continual	Frequent	≤ 60%	> 30%
Moderate Persistent	Daily	≥ 5/month	> 60% to < 80%	> 30%
Mild Persistent	> 2/week	3 to 4/month	≥ 80%	20%-30%
Mild Intermittent	≤ 2/week	≤ 2 nights/month	≥ 80%	< 20%

2007 NHLBI/NAEPP Asthma Guidelines at a Glance

1. Focus on achieving and maintaining control
2. Variability of asthma: Severity considerations
3. Asthma control
   a. Inhaled corticosteroids (ICS) are part of a preferred treatment across all age groups
   b. When stepping up treatment, combination therapy is recommended and long-acting B_2 adrenergic agonist (LABAs) are preferred agents to combine with ICS in patients > 12 years of age.
4. Asthma assessments: Three age groups established
   a. Current impairment considered
   b. Future risk considered

Management

1. Short-acting B_2 adrenergic agonist [SABA (e.g., Albuterol)] for symptom relief or before exercise
2. Daily maintenance with inhaled corticorsteroids [ICS (e.g. Pulmicort, Azmacort, etc.)]
   a. Side effects include candidal infection of the oropharynx, dry mouth, sore throat
3. SABA for symptom breakthrough
4. If symptoms persist, increase inhaled corticosteroids or add a LABA (e.g. Servent); other options include theophylline or antimediators
5. Inhaled anticholingergics (e.g. Atrovent) may be added if necessary
6. Antileukotrienes (Leukotriene receptor antagonist or LTRA) useful in the maintenance of chronic asthma (e.g., Singulair, Accolate)

Specific Step-Wise Management

1. Mild intermittent asthma (exercise-induced bronchospasm or EIB)
   a. SABA for symptom relief or before exercise

        *   Onset within 5 to 15 minutes; peak at 0.5 to 2 hours; duration 3 to 6 hours

2. Mild persistent asthma
   a. Daily maintenance with ICS
   b. Side effects of inhaled steroids include candidal infection of the oropharynx, dry mouth, and sore throat
   c. SABA three times a day or four times a day as needed for symptom breakthrough
   d. If symptoms persist, increase ICS or add long-acting B_2 adrenergic agonist (LABA)
   e. Inhaled anticholinergics may be added if necessary
   f. Antileukotrienes (Leukotriene receptor antagonist/LTRA) useful in the maintenance of chronic asthma induced by allergens, exercise

3. Moderate persistent asthma
   a. Medium dose daily inhaled corticosteroids (ICS) and:
   b. Long acting bronchodilator or:
   c. Oral B2 adrenergic agonist or:
   d. LABA
   e. SABA as needed for breakthrough symptoms

4. Severe Persistent Asthma
   a. High dose inhaled corticosteroids and:
   b. Long-acting bronchodilator and:
   c. Oral corticosteroids
   d. SABA for breakthrough symptoms

Goals of Therapy

1. Minimal or no chronic symptoms day or night
2. Minimal or no exacerbations
3. No limitations on activities; no school missed
4. Maintain (near) normal pulmonary function
5. Minimal use of SABA
6. Minimal or no adverse effects from medications

Asthma Treatment Guideline Rationale

1. Asthma is a chronic airway disease primarily with inflammation and subsequently with smooth muscle dysfunction
2. Even mild asthma is associated with a risk of exacerbations, hospitalizations and irreversible airflow obstruction
3. Anti-inflammatory treatment improves symptoms
4. Asthma is generally undertreated in the U.S.

Asthma Onset or Exacerbation

1. Rules of Twos
   a. More than 2 uses of quick-relief inhaler per week

b.   More than 2 daytime occurrences for asthma symptoms per week
c.   More than 2 nighttime awakenings with asthma symptoms per month
d.   More than 2 quick-relief metered-dose inhaler canisters per year

2. High risk for asthma-related deaths
a.   History of severe exacerbations
    i.   Intensive care
    ii.   Intubation
b.   Two or more hospitalizations a year
c.   Three or more emergency department visits a year
d.   Overuse of inhaled SABAs
    i.   More than 1 canister/month
e.   Poor adherence to treatment plan

Pneumonia

Inflammation of the lower respiratory tract as microorganisms gain access by aspiration, inhalation or hematogenous dissemination

Etiologies by Cohort

1.   Newborns: Group B streptococcus, chlamydia, *E. coli*
2.   Infants and young children < 6 years: Respiratory syncytial virus (RSV), *H. Influenzae, Strep Pneumoniae* [community-acquired pneumonia (CAP)]
3.   Preschool through young adulthood: *Strep pneumoniae, Mycoplasma, chlamydia*
4.   Immunocompromised or malnourished: Pneumocystis carini pneumonia (PCP) or fungi
5.   70 to 80% all pneumonias are viral

Signs/Symptoms

1.   Fever
2.   Shaking chills
3.   Purulent sputum
4.   Lung consolidation on physical exam
5.   Malaise
6.   Pulse oximetry will note decreased oxygenation in severe distress

Differential Diagnoses

1.   Acute bronchitis
2.   Upper respiratory infection (URI)
3.   Cystic fibrosis

Laboratory/Diagnostics

1. Elevated white blood cell (WBC) count; may be low if the patient is immunosuppressed
2. Infiltrates by chest x-ray (CXR)
3. General screening (GS) and culture if indicated
4. CXR and 2 blood cultures minimum if nosocomial
5. Sputum culture warranted if cough is productive

Radiographic Characteristics of Some Bacterial Pneumonias

1. *H. Influenzae*: Lobar consolidation
2. *S. pneumoniae*: Lobar consolidation
3. *Klebsiella*: Lobar consolidation
4. Pneumocystis (PCP): diffuse interstitial, alveolar, apical or upper lobe infiltrates infiltrates
5. *E. coli*: Patchy infiltrates, pleural effusion
6. *Staphylococcus*: Patchy infiltrates
7. *Pseudomonas*: Patchy infiltrates, cavitation

Management of Community Acquired Pneumonia (based on etiology)

1. Pharmacological therapy is based on the infecting organism
    a. Penicillin: *S. pneumoniae*
    b. Macrolides such as azithromycin (Zithromax), clarithromycin (Biaxin), erythromycin, or doxycycline for M. *or Chlamydia pneumoniae*
    c. Amoxicillin or cephalosporin: *H. influenzae*
2. Viral Pneumonia
    a. Supportive measures: Hydration and antipyretics
    b. Antibiotics only if secondary bacterial infections present
    c. Humidified oxygen and chest physiotherapy (PT)
    d. Bronchodilators to improve airway clearance

Cystic Fibrosis

1. An autosomal recessive disorder with a chromosome 7 long arm mutation which produces a defect in epithelial chloride transport resulting in dehydrated, thick secretions
2. A chronic multisystem disorder affecting the respiratory, gastroenterology, hepatobiliary, and reproductive tracts are affected
3. Characterized by recurrent endobronchial infections, progressive obstructive pulmonary disease, and pancreatic insufficiency with intestinal malabsorption
4. Most common in the Caucasian population
5. Life expectancy 30 years

Signs/Symptoms

1.   Viscid meconium in newborn
2.   Recurrent respiratory infection
3.   Large, liquid, bulky, foul stool
4.   Salt-tasting skin
5.   Chronic cough
6.   Barrel chest
7.   Respiratory retraction
8.   Chronic rhinorrhea
9.   Hepatosplenomegaly
10. Fat-soluble vitamin deficiencies
11. Failure to thrive
12. Delayed puberty
13. Infertility

Laboratory/Diagnostics

1.   Pilocarpine iontophoresis sweat test: At least 60 mEq/L chloride in 100 mg of sweat
2.   Pulmonary function tests (PFTs): Obstructive pattern
3.   Hyponatremic, hypochloremic dehydration (alkalosis)
4.   Chest radiograph: Cystic lesions, atelectasis

Management

1.   Referral for specialty management

Sample Questions

1. A 2-month-old presents with a history of upper-respiratory infection symptoms for several days, a decrease in appetite, tachypnea, and paroxysmal wheezing. The most likely diagnosis is:
    a. Asthma
    b. Bronchiolitis
    c. Bacterial Pneumonmia
    d. Croup

2. The National Asthma Education and Prevention Program states there is a stepwise approach for treating asthma, with 4 levels to classify the severity of the disease. A 10-year-old child's symptoms occur 4 times a week during the day and 3 times during the night, with an FEV1 of 80%. What would be the severity?
    a. Severe persistent
    b. Moderate persistent
    c. Mild persistent
    d. Mild intermittent

3. The nurse practitioner is discussing home maintenance with a metered-dose inhaler (MDI). All of the following are true except:
    a. Breathe the medication mist in deeply, and hold your breath to the count of 10
    b. Shake the canister while taking a deep breath in and out
    c. The MDI should not be used with antileukotrienes.
    d. Report the use of quick-release inhalers more than 2 times per week

Answers

1. Correct Answer: B
These are symptoms of bronchiolitis, which are usually manifested in the winter and fall months. It is most commonly caused by a viral illness such as respiratory syncytial virus or adenoviruses. Croup has a characteristic barking cough. Asthma is characterized by inflammation, and wheezing can be triggered by allergens.

2. Correct Answer: C
Symptoms of mild persistent asthma include symptoms occurring greater than 2 times a week during the day and greater than 2 times a month during the night. The forced expiratory volume in 1 second is greater than 80%.

3. Correct Answer: C
Proper use of the MDI includes shaking the canister prior to use. This may be easily done while taking a deep breath in and out. The canister should be depressed at the beginning of the next breath, and the medication mist should be breathed in deeply. Hold the breath to count of 10. Antileukotrtienes are useful in the maintenance of chronic asthma and increase use or need of an inhaler should be reported to the practitioner.

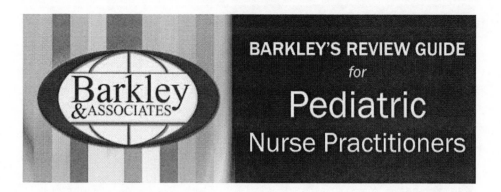

Inflammatory Musculoskeletal Issues and Disorders

Osgood-Schlatter Diseases

Inflammation of the tibial tubercle as a result of repetitive stressors (e.g., avulsion injury) in patients with immature skeletal development

1. Peak ages: 11 to 14 years
2. Associated with rapid growth spurt

Signs/Symptoms

1. Pain and tenderness at tibial tubercle
2. Point tenderness
3. Enlargement compared to unaffected side

Laboratory/Diagnostic

1. None; typically, this is a diagnosis that that is made clinically
2. Radiographs to rule out more serious causes of pain

Management

1. Self-limiting disease
2. Limit activity to control pain
3. Complete activity restriction is not recommended
4. Knee immobilizers may provide some relief

Toxic Synovitis

Self-limiting inflammation of the hip, most likely due to a viral or immune cause

1. Occurs most often in children ages 2 to 6 years old but can occur from ages one to 15 years
2. Affects males more often than females

Signs/Symptoms

1. Painful limp
2. Unilateral involvement
3. Insidious onset

4. Internal rotation of hip causes spasm
5. No obvious inspection/palpation signs

Laboratory/Diagnostics

1. Normal radiographs
2. Normal joint fluid aspiration

Management

1. Analgesics
2. Bed rest as needed
3. Typically benign and self-limiting
4. Hospitalization should be considered if the patient has a high fever or septic arthritis is suspected
5. It is very important to investigate a child with a limp

Legg-Calve-Perthes Disease (LCPD)

Aseptic or avascular necrosis of the femoral head

Etiology/Incidence

1. Unknown etiology, possibly due to vascular disruption
2. Slightly shorter stature or delayed bone age compared to peers
3. Most common in Caucasian boys, ages 4 to 9 years
4. 15% bilateral

Signs/Symptoms

1. Insidious onset of limp with knee pain
2. Pain may also accur in groin or lateral hip
3. Pain less acute and severe than transient synovitis or septic arthritis
4. Afebrile

Physical Findings

1. Limited passive internal rotation and abduction of the hip joint
2. May be resisted by mild spasm or guarding
3. Hip flexion contracture and leg muscle atrophy occur in long-standing cases

Differential Diagnoses

1. Transient synovitis
2. Septic arthritis
3. Hematogenous osteomyelitis
4. Various types of hemoglobinopathy
5. Hypothyroidism
6. Epiphyseal dysplasia

Laboratory/Diagnostics

1.   Radiograph studies
    a.   Notes disease progress and sphericity of femoral head
    b.   Used initially for definitive diagnosis
    c.   Subsequently used to assess reparative process
2.   No labs necessary

Management/Treatment

1.   Goal: To restore range of motion (ROM) while maintaining femoral head within acetabulum
2.   Observation only
    a.   If full range of motion (FROM) is preserved
    b.   Less than 6 years of age
    c.   Involvement of less than one-half of the femoral head
3.   Aggressive treatment
    a.   Indicated when more than one-half femoral head is involved and in children older than 6 years
    b.   Use orthosis
        i.   To produce abduction with or without internal rotation
        ii.   Document containment with radiograph
        iii.   Worn until early ossification noted
    c.   Activity permissible while in brace
4.   Surgical Treatment
    a.   Femoral osteotomy (shelf procedure)
    b.   Used more commonly as an alternative to orthosis
5.   Child/Family Education
    a.   Inform family that legg-calve-perthes disease lasts 1 to 3 years
    b.   Potentially serious if not treated properly

Slipped Capital Femoral Ephiphysis (SCFE)

Spontaneous dislocation of femoral head (capital epiphysis) both downward and backward relative to the femoral neck and secondary to disruption of the epiphyseal plate

Etiology/Incidence

1.   Etiology: Unknown; perhaps precipitated by puberty-related hormone changes
2.   Generally occurs without severe, sudden force or trauma but is sometimes related to trauma
3.   Typical during growth spurt and prior to menarche in girls
4.   Rare: 1:100,000 to 8:100,000
5.   More common in males and African American adolescents
6.   Bilateral involvement 25 to 33%; 1 side follows the other

7.   Incidence is greater among obese adolescents with sedentary lifestyles

Signs/Symptoms

1.   Varies with acuity
2.   Most have a limp
3.   Varying degrees of aching and pain noted in the groin and often referred to thigh and/or knee
4.   When acute, severe pain with the inability to ambulate or move hip is noted
5.   Physical findings
       a.   Unable to properly flex hip as femur abducts/rotates externally
       b.   May observe limb shortening, resulting from proximal displacement of metaphysic

Differential Diagnosis

1.   Knee complaint with no obvious cause
2.   Trauma
3.   Septic arthritis
4.   Transient (e.g., toxic synovitis)
5.   Juvenile arthritis
6.   LCPD

Laboratory/Diagnostics

1.   Accurate history combined with knowledge of etiological factors
2.   Radiographs
       a.   Confirms diagnosis
       b.   Shows degree of slipping between femoral head and neck
3.   Laboratory studies
       a.   Depend on findings from physical exam and history
       b.   Done to rule out associated causes of infection or inflammation

Management/Treatment

1.   Immediate referral to orthopedist
2.   Treatment goal is to prevent further slippage
3.   No ambulation permitted
4.   Surgery
       a.   Pin fixation with open epiphysiodesis using a bone graft
       b.   For stabilization of the upper femur and causes growth plate to close
5.   Monitor other hip for same problem

Genu Varum (Bowleg)

Lateral bowing of the tibia, often due to joint laxity; considered a normal variant until age 2

Signs/Symptoms

1.   Lateral bowing up to 20 degrees is normal until 24 months
2.   Normal bowing does not increase after walking
3.   Retains full range of motion

Laboratory/Diagnostics

1.   None indicated for typical bowing
2.   May be used to evaluate extreme or unilateral bowing

Management

1.   None necessary under age two if appears as normal variant
2.   Needs further evaluation if:
        a.   Continues after age 2
        b.   Unilateral
        c.   Becomes progressively worse after first year

Genu Valgum (Knock-Knee)

Knees are abnormally close and ankle space is increased; typically evolves to normal alignment by age 7 years

Signs/Symptoms

1.   Knees close together
2.   Distance between medial malleoli is more than 3 inches
3.   No pain
4.   FROM
5.   Walk or run may be awkward

Laboratory/Diagnostics

1.   None necessary
2.   Radiographs if over age 7 or if unilateral involvement is present

Management

1.   None necessary
2.   Normal variant in children under 7 years old
3.   Older children need further evaluation

Scoliosis

1.   Lateral curvature of the spine is most common in adolescence

2. Other types are congenital (e.g., infancy) or neuromuscular (associated with conditions)
3. Most cases are idiopathic
4. Occurs more often in females with an 8:1 ratio, with a family history in 70% of cases

Signs/Symptoms

1. Alteration in back contour
2. May occur any age
3. Rarely painful
4. Asymmetry of shoulder height and scapulae
5. Uneven hip and waistline
6. Rib asymmetry

Laboratory/Diagnostics

1. Adam's forward bending test
   a. Bend forward 90 degrees with knees straight and arms hanging down
   b. Observe for abnormal prominence of scapulae, thoracic ribs, hip, etc.
2. Radiographs for further evaluation

Management

1. Further evaluation in any degree if pain occurs
2. If no pain exist and if less than 25 degrees curvature
   a. No further evaluation is needed if skeletally mature
3. In younger children, bracing is 80% successful
   a. Curves more than 40 degrees
   b. Surgery for lumbar curve more than 40 degrees or throracic curve more than 50 degrees
4. Cardio-pulmonary restriction may occur in curves more than 75 degrees

Developmental Dysplasia of the Hip (DDH)

Abnormal dislocation of the hip in which the femoral head is partially or completely displaced from the acetabulum

1. May be congenital but not detected until ambulation
2. Occurs more often in girls and on the left side
3. Incidence is 1.5:1,000 live births
4. Caucasians are at increased risk
5. Causes are multifactorial and include intrauterine and genetic factors

Signs/Symptoms

1. Physical examination is critical

2.   Often detected with newborn exam but not always
3.   If not detected at birth, a limp may be noticed when infant begins walking
4.   Painless
5.   Decreased hip abduction in older children
6.   Infant signs:
       a.   Galeazzi's sign
           i.   Compare knee height with infant supine, hips and knees flexed
           ii.   Asymmetry suggests DDH
           iii.   Not helpful if DDH is bilateral
       b.   Barlow's sign:
           i.   Movement of the femoral head can be felt as it slips out of posterior acetabulum
       c.   Ortolani's sign
           i.   Click as felt or heart as the femoral head enters and exits acetabulum
           ii.   In the older infant, decreased abduction is more significant

Laboratory/Diagnostics

1.   Radiographs after 6 months of age
2.   Ultrasound may be used

Management

1.   Less than 6 months old: Stabilization
2.   More than 6 months old: Surgical reduction

Muscular Dystrophy

Progressive genetic disorder beginning in the lower extremities and progressing to the upper extremities and torso

1.   The most common inherited neuromuscular disease in children
2.   Affects 1:3,500 males
3.   Average age of diagnosis is 3 to 5 years

Signs/Symptoms

1.   Abnormalities of gait and posture
2.   Developmental clumsiness
3.   Cannot keep up with developing peers
4.   Gower's maneuver
       a.   Child "walks" hands up legs to attain standing position when getting up
       b.   Suggests pelvic girdle weakness
       c.   May occur in other conditions

5. Depressed proximal muscle strength
6. Wheelchair dependent by age 12
7. Contractures as joint mobility is lost
8. Kyphoscoliosis
9. Eventual death from cardiopulmonary failure

Laboratory/Diagnostics

1. Creatine kinase: Markedly elevated in affected males (15,000 to 35,000 IU/L)
2. Electromyography (EMG): Myopathy
3. ECG: Tall R waves in right precordium, deep Q in left precordium and limb leads
4. Muscle biopsy: Necrotic degenerating fibers present; dystrophic immunoreactivity confirms diagnosis
5. DNA analysis of gene

Management

1. Symptomatic care
2. Delay progression
3. Strength and mobility
4. Refer family for genetic testing

Ankle Sprain

Stretching and/or tearing of the ligaments around the ankle, typically involving the lateral ligament complex

1. Most common sports injury
2. Most common musculoskeletal injury
3. Usually a forced inversion (lateral ankle) or eversion (medial ankle)

Signs/Symptoms

1. Grade I: Stretching but no tearing of ligament; no joint instability
   a. Local tenderness
   b. Minimal edema
   c. Ecchymoses typically insignificant or absent
   d. Full range of motion remains although may be uncomfortable
   e. Patient retains weight bearing ability
2. Grade II: Partial (incomplete) tearing of ligament; some joint instability but definite end-point to laxity
   a. Pain immediately upon injury
   b. Localized edema and eccymoses
   c. Significant pain with weight bearing
   d. Range of motion is limited

3.   Grade III: Complete ligamentous tearing; joint unstable with no definite endpoint to ligamentous stressing
   a.   Severe pain immediately upon injury
   b.   Significant edema along foot and ankle
   c.   Profound ecchymoses due to hemorrhage: Worsens over several days
   d.   Patient cannot weight bear
   e.   No range of motion to ankle

Laboratory/Diagnostic

1.   Radiograph is indicated according to Ottawa Ankle Rule
2.   Also indicated if:
   a.   There is pain near the malleoli and
   b.   Bone tenderness is present at the posterior edge of the distal 6 cm or the tip of either malleolus or:
   c.   The patient is unable to bear weight for at least four steps at the time of injury and evaluation
3.   Otherwise diagnostic studies not indicated

Management

1.   **R**est: Weight bearing should be avoided for the first several days
2.   **I**ce: Should be applied on top of the compression dressing as quickly as possible following injury, 30 minutes on and off alternately
3.   **C**ompression: Immediate secure compression will minimize edema and support stability of the ankle
4.   **E**levation: For several days following injury reduces pain and swelling and promotes recovery
   a.   All grades including III (unless severe grade III) respond well to rest, ice, compression and elevation (**RICE**)
5.   Nonsteroidal anti-inflammatory drugs (NSAIDs) for pharmacologic relief

Sample Questions

1. A genetic disorder that is characterized by blue sclera, triangular faces, and hearing loss is:

    a. Rhett boney syndrome
    b. Osteogenesis imperfecta
    c. Femoral retroversion bilaterally
    d. Valgum syndrome

2. A provider is examining a new patient who is 2 months old and when first examining the baby, she notices that one leg appears shorter than the other. The provider knows when measuring regions that appear asymmetric, she should:

    a. Use a ruler in inches
    b. Measure in centimeters always
    c. Use an anatomical landmark
    d. Use a string around the extremity, and then place it on a ruler

3. A mother brings her daughter to the clinic with the complaint that she cannot keep up with the other children at preschool. She states that her daughter can't run as well and often falls. You notice that her daughter, who was sitting on the carpet, "walks" her hands up her legs to attain a standing position when getting up. As a result, you suspect:

    a. Legg-Calve-Perthes disease
    b. Muscular dystrophy
    c. Slipped capital femoral epiphysis
    d. Osgood-Schlatter disease

Answers

1. Correct Answer: B

Osteogenesis imperfecta characteristics include: bones fracture easily, can usually be traced through the family, near normal stature or slightly shorter, blue sclera (the normally white area of the eye), dental problems, and eventual hearing loss.

2. Correct Answer: C

Limb length discrepancy can be measured by a provider during a physical examination and through x-rays. Usually, the practitioner measures the level of the hips as the anatomical landmark when the child is standing barefoot.

3. Correct Answer: B

Muscular dystrophy is a progressive genetic disorder beginning in the lower extremities and progressing to the upper extremities and torso. It is the most common inherited neuromuscular disease in children. The average age of diagnosis is 3 to 5 years. Classic features include: Abnormalities of gait and posture, developmental clumsiness, inability to keep up with developing peers, and Gower's maneuver. With Gower's maneuver, the child "walks" hands up legs to attain a standing position when getting up. This suggests pelvic girdle weakness but may occur in other conditions

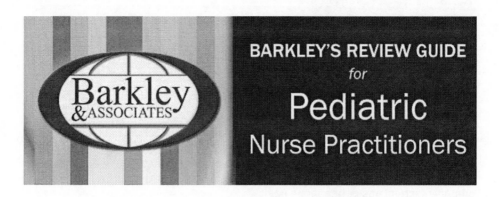

Neurological Issues and Disorders

Cranial Nerves

Number	Name	Major Functions	Type
CN I:	Olfactory	Smell	S = Some
CN II:	Optic	Vision	S = Say
CN III:	Oculomotor	Most EOMs, opening eyelids, papillary constriction	M = Marry
CN IV:	Trochlear	Down and inward eye movement	M = Money
CN V:	Trigeminal	Muscles of mastication; sensation of face, scalp, cornea, mucus membranes and nose	B = But
CN VI:	Abducens	Lateral eye movement	M = My
CN VII:	Facial	Move face, close mouth & eyes, taste (anterior 2/3), saliva & tear secretion	B = Brother
CN VIII:	Acoustic	Hearing & equilibrium	S = Says
CN IX:	Glossopharyngeal	Phonation, one-third), gag reflex, carotid reflex swallowing, taste (posterior	B = Betty
CN X:	Vagus	Talking, swallowing, general sensation from the carotid body, carotid reflex	B = Boop
CN XI:	Spinal accessory	Movement of trapezius & sternomastoid muscles (shrug shoulders)	M = Marilyn
CN XII:	Hypoglossal	Moves the tongue	M = Monroe

"**O**n **O**ld **O**lympus **T**owering **T**ops **A** **F**in **A**nd **G**erman **V**iewed **S**ome **H**ops"

Headache

Although headache in itself is not actually a disease entity, it is discussed separately because it is a very common complaint among school-aged and adolescent children. Such headaches may present for a multitude of reasons and can be difficult to evaluate. Proper evaluation of the history of the headache, and associated symptoms, are essential to making an accurate diagnosis. There are 4 primary mechanisms of headache pain:

1.　　Vascular dilation:　Distention of pain-sensitive cranial arteries. This is the mechanism of pain behind migraine, fever, vasodilator drugs, metabolic disturbance or systemic infection. It is typically seen in school-aged and particularly adolescent patients.
2.　　Muscular contraction:　Contraction of head and neck muscles; may be involved as cause of pain in tension or psychogenic headache
3.　　Traction:　Traction of pain-sensitive structures; brain tumors, mass lesions, abscess, hematoma, increased intracranial pressure (ICP)
4.　　Inflammation:　Inflammation of pain-sensitive areas, such as the meninges, sinuses, and teeth

Components of Headache Evaluation

For symptom assessment, use the OLD CART system:　Onset, Location, Duration, Characteristics, Aggravating factors, Remedial/Alleviating factors, and Treatment ("What was done and did it work?")

1.　　Chronology is the most important history item
2.　　Location, duration and quality should be evaluated
3.　　Associated activity:　Exertion, sleep, tension, and relaxation
4.　　Timing of the menstrual cycle
5.　　Presence of associated symptoms
6.　　Presence of "triggers"

First or Worst Headaches

Need to rule out potentially life threatening or serious etiologies:

Febrile Patient

1.　　Meningitis:　Bacterial, viral, tuberculous, aseptic
2.　　Brain abscess or other intracranial infection
3.　　Encephalitis
4.　　Sinusitis
5.　　Associated infection; strep throat, influenza, mono, rubeola

Risk for Meningitis with Fever

1.　　Enteroviral meningitis occurs in 10% to 30% of febrile infants
2.　　Frequency of bacterial meningitis is 1% to 2%

   a.   It is present in 10% to 14% of infants with temperatures higher
         than 101.8°F (38.8°C)
   b.   Causative agents include: Group *B streptococcus, S.
         pneumoniae, H. influenzae, Salmonella, N. meningitidis*, protozoa
         and *E. coli*
3.   Infants between 6 to 12 months are at the highest risk
4.   90% of cases occur in children ages 1 month to 5 years

Signs/Symptoms

Most are behavioral responses

1.   Newborns and Young Infants
      a.   Mimics septicemia
      b.   Temperature instability
      c.   Respiratory distress
      d.   Irritability, lethargy
      e.   Poor feeding
      f.   Vomiting
      g.   Bulging fontanel
      h.   Increased ICP
      i.   No stiff neck
2.   Older Infants and children
      a.   Nausea and vomiting
      b.   Irritability, confusion
      c.   Anorexia
      d.   Headaches, back pain, nuchal rigidity
      e.   Hyperesthesia, cranial nerve palsy, ataxia
      f.   Photophobia
      g.   Positive Kernig's sign
            i.   Flexion of the legs 90 degrees at hip
            ii.   Pain on extension of leg
      h.   Positive Brudzinski's sign
            i.   Involuntary flexion of legs when neck is flexed
      i.   Headache with increased ICP

Diagnostic Tests

1.   Cerebrospinal fluid (CSF) analysis via lumbar puncture
      a.   Cloudy
      b.   Increased cell count (300 to 10,000)
      c.   Increased protein
      d.   Decreased glucose

Afebrile Patient

1.   Subarachnoid hemorrhage
2.   Intraparenchymal hemorrhage

3.   Postictal headache
4.   Cerebral ischemia
5.   Severe hypertension
6.   Acute dental disease
7.   Acute glaucoma, inflammatory disease of the eye/orbit

Brain Tumors

1.   Etiology is unknown
        a.   May be genetic predisposition
        b.   Congenital factors
        c.   Environmental exposures
2.   Two most common primary tumors
        a.   Cerebellar astorcytomas: 10 to 20%
        b.   Medulloblastoma
3.   Infratentorial tumors predominate: 4 to 11 years of age

Signs/Symptoms

1.   Infants:
        a.   Increased head circumference, tense bulging fontanel
        b.   Irritability
        c.   Head tilt
        d.   Loss of developmental milestones
2.   Older Children
        a.   Headache
                i.   Worst in the morning followed by vomiting
                ii.   Usually increases in frequency
        b.   Abnormal neurologic or ocular examination
                i.   Two to 4 months after headaches
                ii.   Specific neurologic symptoms may occur later: Possible localized central nervous system (CNS) tumor?
                iii.   Ataxia, hemiparesis, cranial nerve palsies
                iv.   Somnolence
                v.   Seizures
                vi.   Head tilt, failure to thrive (FTT), diabetes insipidus
                vii.   Nuchal rigidity, papilledema
                viii.   Uncoordinated or clumsy
                ix.   Poor fine motor control
                x.   Positive Babinski's sign
                xi.   Behavioral changes

Diagnostic Tests

1.   Magnetic resonance imaging (MRI)
2.   Computed axial tomography (CT scan)
3.   Angiography

4.   Lumbar puncture (LP)

Migraine Headaches (Vascular Headaches)

Migraine headaches are divided into two categories, classic migraine (migraine with aura) and common migraine (migraine without aura). Migraines have been related to dilation and excessive pulsation of branches of the external carotid artery

Causes/Incidence

1.   Common migraine < 10 years of age at onset
2.   Classic migraine onset > 10 years of age
3.   Often there is a family history
4.   Females more often affected than males
5.   A variety of "triggers" are associated with migraine: Emotional or physical stress, lack or excess sleep, missed meals, specific foods, alcoholic beverages, menstruation, use of oral contraceptives
6.   Nitrate containing foods
7.   Changes in weather
8.   History of motion sickness or cyclic vomiting is common

Symptoms

1.   Unilateral, lateralized throbbing headache that occurs episodically (common may be bilateral)
2.   May be dull or throbbing
3.   Build up gradually and last for several hours or longer
4.   Focal neurologic disturbances may precede or accompany migraines (classic migraine)
5.   Visual disturbances occur commonly: field defects, luminous visual hallucinations (i.e., stars, sparks or zigzag of lights)
6.   Aphasia, numbness, tingling, clumsiness or weakness may occur
7.   Nausea and vomiting
8.   Photophobia and phonophobia

Variant Migraine Syndromes

1.   Hemiplegic migraine: Presents with hemiplegia, aphasia, speech disturbances followed by headache and associated symptoms; headache contralateral to hemiplegia; headache less symptomatic than hemiplegia
2.   Confusional migraine: More common in younger children; period of confusion and disorientation followed by vomiting and deep sleep, waking feeling well; headache may not be described
3.   Abdominal migraine: Episodic abdominal pain with nausea, vomiting followed or accompanied by headache

4. Basilar migraine: Dizziness, vertigo, syncope, and dysarthria preceding variable headaches and vomiting

Physical Exam Findings

1. Many times findings are normal although may see neurological deficits as described above
2. Appears ill
3. Careful neuro exam for focal deficits or findings supportive of tumor

Laboratory/Diagnostics

1. In patients with new migraine headaches, a variety of baseline studies must be done to rule out organic causes
2. Blood chemistries, basic metabolic panel (BMP)
3. Complete blood count test (CBC)
4. Venereal Disease Research Laboratory test (VDRL)
5. Erythrocyte sedimentation rate (ESR): Medical test for inflammation
6. CT scan of the head
7. Other studies as indicated by the history and physical exam

Management

1. Avoidance of trigger factors is very important; have the patient keep a headache diary
2. Improve general health: Balanced diet, aerobic exercise, regular sleep
3. Relaxation/stress management techniques (e.g., counseling, biofeedback)
4. Eliminate monosodium glutamate (MSG) and nitrates or nitrites from diet
5. Stabilize or wean caffeine intake
6. Prophylactic therapy if attacks occur more than 3 to 4 times per month, or if migraines interfere with daily functioning or school; for example,
   a. Non-steroidal anti-inflammatory drugs (NSAIDs) in chronic, low doses daily
   b. Propanolol (Inderal): < 35 kg: 10 to 20 mg by mouth, three times a day; if > 35 kg: 20 to 40 mg by mouth, three times a day
   c. Amitriptyline (Elavil): 25 to 50 mg/dose by mouth at bedtime
   d. Imipramine (Tofranil): 10 to 150 mg daily
   e. Clonidine (Catapres): 0.2 to 0.6 mg daily
   f. Verapamil (Calan): 15 to 30 mg/kg/24 hour by mouth twice a day

This is not an all-inclusive list. Various ergotamines, anticonvulsants, monoamine oxidase (MAO) inhibitors, and antiserotonin drugs are also used for prophylaxis of migraine.

Management of Acute Attack

1. Rest in a dark, quiet room

2.   A simple analgesic (NSAID) (e.g., naproxen, ketorolac) taken right away may provide some relief
3.   Antiemetics (e.g., metoclopramide): 1 to 2 mg/kg/dose every 2 to 6 hours
4.   Sumatriptan (Imitrex): 6 mg subcutaneous at onset, may repeat in one hour, to a total of 3 times per day
5.   Sumatriptan (Imitrex): 25 mg orally at onset of headache; if no relief in 2 hours, give 25 to 100 mg every 2 hours up to a daily dose of 200 mg
    a.   Maximum single dose: 100 mg/dose
    b.   Nasal: 5 to 20 mg/dose into one nostril or divided into each nostril
    c.   If headache returns, dose may be repeated in 2 hour up to a maximum of 40 mg/24 hours
6.   Cafergot: 1 mg at onset of migraine attack, then 1 mg every 30 minutes as needed, up to a maximum of 3 mg

Seizure Disorder

A transient disturbance of cerebral function due to an abnormal paroxysmal neuronal discharge in the brain, resulting in a variety of clinical signs and symptoms that may or may not involve a loss of consciousness

1.   There are several types of seizures, each with different presentations, diagnostic findings, and treatments
2.   The term epilepsy denotes any disorder characterized by recurrent seizures

Causes/Incidence

1.   Affects approximately 0.5% of the overall population in the United States
2.   Epilepsy is the second most common neurological disorder
3.   Congenital abnormalities and perinatal injuries may result in seizures presenting in infancy and early childhood
4.   Metabolic disorders: Hypocalcemia, hypoglycemia, pyridoxine deficiency, renal failure, acidosis and others
5.   Trauma is an important cause in adolescents
6.   Tumors and other space occupying lesions
7.   Infectious diseases: Bacterial meningitis, herpes encephalitis, neurosyphilis

Seizure Categories

Partial

Focal origin: One hemisphere

1.   Simple partial seizures
    a.   No loss of consciousness
    b.   Focal motor symptoms (convulsive jerking)

        c.   Speech arrest or vocalizations
        d.   Jacksonian march
        e.   May exhibit special sensory symptoms: Light flashes, buzzing
        f.   May exhibit autonomic symptoms: Sweating, flushing
        g.   Lasts approximately 1 minute

2.   Complex partial seizures
        a.   Impaired consciousness (> 20 seconds) before, during or after the symptoms described above, starting as a staring episode then progressing to impairment of consciousness
        b.   With or without automatisms; symptoms noted in simple partial seizure category

Generalized Seizures

Bilateral, involving both hemispheres

1.   Absence (petit mal)
        a.   Brief "staring" episodes (10 to 20 seconds)
        b.   Onset and termination are very brief
        c.   Almost always begin in childhood

2.   Myoclonic
        a.   Brief, sudden muscle contractions generalized or localized, symmetric or asymmetric, synchronous or asynchronous
        b.   Sometimes with mild clonic, tonic or atonic components; occasionally autonomic components

3.   Clonic
        a.   Sustained rhythmic jerking of a portion of the body
        b.   Loss or impairment of consciousness

4.   Tonic
        a.   Sudden increase in muscle tone producing a number of characteristic postures
        b.   Consciousness is usually partially or completely lost
        c.   Postictal alteration of consciousness is usually brief; may last several minutes

5.   Tonic-clonic (grand mal)
        a.   Sudden loss of consciousness with arrested respirations
        b.   The clonic phase involves increased muscle tone followed by bilateral rhythmic jerks lasting 2 to 3 minutes, followed by flaccid coma
        c.   Urinary and or fecal incontinence may occur
        d.   The postictal state is characterized by deep sleep for up to an hour, headache, disorientation, muscle discomfort and nausea; can last minutes to hours

6.   Atonic
        a.   Sudden loss of muscle tone

b.   May result in head drop or falling to the ground

An eyewitness account is extremely helpful and should be obtained whenever possible.

Laboratory/Diagnostics

1.   Investigate the underlying cause
2.   Seizure assessment includes the following:
      a.   Presence of aura
      b.   Onset
      c.   Spread
      d.   Type of movement
      e.   Body parts involved
      f.   Pupil changes and reactivity
      g.   Duration
      h.   Loss/level of consciousness
      i.   Incontinence
      j.   Behavioral and neurological changes after session of seizure activity
3.   Complete blood count test (CBC) with differential, glucose, renal function tests, liver function tests, and a serologic test for syphilis should be performed
4.   Other tests to rule out suspected etiology as indicated by the history and age of the patient (e.g., CT scan, lumbar puncture, CT or MRI of the head for all new onset seizures)
5.   Electroencephalogram (EEG): Most important test to determine seizure classification

Management: Acute Attack

1.   Initial management is supportive as most seizures are self-limiting
      a.   Maintain open airway
      b.   Protect patient from injuries
      c.   Administer oxygen if patient is cyanotic
2.   Do not force artificial airways or objects between teeth
3.   Parental anticonvulsants are used to stop convulsive seizures rapidly
      a.   Lorazapam (Ativan) OR
      b.   Bezodiazepines (Valium)

Treatment

Decision to treat is based on several considerations
1.   Probability of recurrence
      a.   One-time seizure usually not treated
      b.   60% of newly diagnosed children will enter remission upon treatment

        c.   40% of cases are either intractable or refractory to anti-epileptic medications or treated with unacceptable side effects

        d.   Recurrent seizures: Indication for treatment

        e.   Probability of death (most common with uncontrolled, nocturnal, generalized tonic-clonic seizures)

2.   Pharmacological Treatment

        a.   Goal:

                i.   Appropriate match of drug to specific type of seizure

                ii.   Control of seizures with minimal side effects

                iii.   Improves quality of life

                iv.   Promotes optimal growth and development

        b.   Anti-epileptic medications: Pharmacodynamics/pharmacokinetics

                i.   Augment inhibitory processes or oppose excitatory ones

                ii.   Directly affect specific ion channels

                iii.   Indirectly influence synthesis, metabolism, or function of neurotransmitters

                iv.   Indirectly affect receptors that control channel opening and closing

                v.   Prescribed by weight in kilograms and titrated to achieve therapeutic levels

                vi.   Monitor serum drug level (morning trough only) and alter dosages accordingly in the initial phase of treatment

                vii.   Monitor CBC and liver function tests (LFTs) after therapeutic levels have been achieved, then as needed

                viii.   Routine serum monitoring is not cost effective and not recommended, unless:

                        1.   Child and family is noncompliant

                        2.   Status epilepticus occurs

3.   Child/adolescent experiencing a growth spurt

4.   Child receiving more than one drug

5.   Change in type, duration or frequency of seizures

6.   Signs and symptoms of toxicity

7.   Child has hepatic or renal disease

8.   Child has cognitive or physical disabilities

        a.   Pharmacologic choice depends upon type of seizure

                i.   Broad Spectrum:

                        1.   Phenytoin (Dilantin)

                        2.   Primidone (Mysoline)

                        3.   Valproate (Depakote)

                ii.   Partial Seizures:

                        1.   Cabamazepine (Tegretol)

                        2.   Gabapentin (Neurontin)

                        3.   Levetiracetam (Keppra)

                        4.   Oxcarbazepine (Trileptal)

5.   Topiramate (Topomax)
9.   Zonisamide (Zonegran)
    a.   Weaning off anticonvulsants: Should be done over a 3-to-6-month period; can be done after a minimum of 2 seizure-free years, a normal EEG, and unchanged physical examination

Miscellaneous Associated Manifestations and Concerns

1.   Seizures (depending on type, severity, age of onset) can have profound negative effects on growth and development; however, supportive family environments can play a positive moderating role
2.   Cognitive function:
    a.   Most patients demonstrate normal intelligence
    b.   Low-severity seizures: Average school performance
    c.   High-severity seizure: Are at risk for cognitive dysfunction
3.   Mental health co-morbidity
    a.   50% of patients may have co-morbid psychiatric disorder
    b.   Anxiety disorders: Most common
    c.   Presence of a mood disorder (depression)
    d.   Presence of aggression and violence as a post-ictal psychosis phenomenon
4.   Growth: Weight gain or loss depending upon the medications and/or concomitant disorders
5.   Behavioral problems
    a.   Related
    b.   Deficient family mastery of a chronic condition
    c.   Low parental confidence in managing discipline
6.   Injury potential
    a.   No swimming alone
    b.   No climbing trees
    c.   Unable to drive if seizures are uncontrolled (length of time varies by state)

Referral

Refer when:

1.   Seizures continue despite therapeutic monitoring through anticonvulsant levels
2.   Regression of developmental skills occurs
3.   Regression of cognitive function occurs
4.   Side effect profile is unacceptable

Primary Care Follow-Up

1.   Monitor growth
2.   Monitor developmental milestones

3.   Safety updates at each well child check (WCC) visit: Tailored to the child's age/development and severity of seizures
4.   Immunizations
5.   Adolescent issues:
    a.   Noncompliance with medications and safety issues
    b.   Some anticonvulsants can lower the effects of oral contraceptives
    c.   Pregnancy: Genetic counseling should be recommended
    d.   Teratogenicity with high anticonvulsant doses and or polytherapy

Long-Term Implications

1.   Good: Remission with or without treatment
2.   Poor prognosis:
    a.   High initial seizure density
    b.   Etiology of metabolic disorder

Febrile Seizures

Seizures occurring during the course of and as a result of fever

1.   Occur in 5% of children, peak incidence between 1 and 3 years of age
2.   Risk factors include a family history of seizure disorder, tobacco use by mother during pregnancy, prematurity, neonatal hospitalization > 28 days, and/or frequent infections in the first year
3.   If a seizure occurs > 24 hours after fever onset, it is likely due to infection

Signs/Symptoms

1.   Majority are tonic-clonic
2.   15% may be myoclonic
3.   Most episodes last < 5 minutes
4.   Physical exam to rule out infectious cause of seizure
5.   Emphasis on ruling out meningitis
    a.   Neonates: Nonspecific signs (e.g., lethargy, poor feeding, irritability)
    b.   Infants/Toddlers: Bulging fontanelle, high pitched cry, vomiting, irritability
    c.   Classic signs of meningitis in children > 2 years of age: Headache, nuchal rigidity, and vomiting

Laboratory/Diagnostics

1.   Lumbar puncture if meningitis is suspected
2.   EEG, chemistries, and serologies are not indicated

Management

1.   Protect airway; place in side-lying position
2.   Lorazepam intravenously

3.   Sponge baths
4.   Acetaminophen
5.   Phenobarbital or valproic acid prophylaxis only if:
      a.   Family history of seizures
      b.   Prior abnormal neurological exam
      c.   Seizure with focal component
      d.   More than one seizure in 24 hours
6.   Recurrence rate

Neurofibromatosis (Vonrecklinghausen Disease)

A neurocutaneous syndrome characterized by numerous café-au-lait spots on the body and nerve tumors on the skin and in the body

1.   Progressive disorder, does not affect intelligence
2.   Occurs in 1 in 4,000 persons
3.   Autosomal dominant, associated with chromosome 17
4.   Severity is highly variable

Signs/Symptoms

1.   Multiple café-au-lait Coffin-Lowry syndrome (CLS) spots as noted
2.   The child may be developmentally delayed
3.   Seizures
4.   Diagnostic criteria: Must have at least 2
      a.   Six or more CLS spots > 5 mm in prepubertal child or > 15 mm postpubertal
      b.   Two or more cutaneous, or a sufficient quantity of neurofibromas, or 1 plexiform neurofibroma
      c.   Axillary or inguinal freckling
      d.   Two or more iris Lisch nodules
      e.   Distinctive osseous lesions
      f.   First degree relative

Laboratory/Diagnostics

1.   Slit-lamp exam for ocular involvement
2.   Cranial MRI for gliomas
3.   Radiographs: Osseous lesions, other tumors
4.   EEG
5.   Psychologic evaluation
6.   Audiogram

Management

1.   Manage sequelae
      a.   Constipation
      b.   Seizures

      c.   Learning disabilities
2.   Surgical debulking
3.   Correct scoliosis

Tic Disorders

Brief, abrupt, nonpurposeful movements or utterances

1.   The most common is Tourette's syndrome
2.   Movements usually involve the face, neck, or shoulders and sometimes, muscles of the limbs or other parts of the body
3.   Other psychobehavioral problems, including attention deficit hyperactivity disorder (ADHD) and obsessive-compulsive behaviors, are also associated with Tourette's syndrome, although not all children with Tourette's syndrome display these problems

Etiology and Incidence

1.   Frequently unrecognized as a movement disorder in children
2.   Onset is between 6 and 12 years of age but can be seen as late as age 21
3.   Cause is unknown
4.   Occurs in multiple generations within families
5.   The prevalence is higher in males than females

Predisposing Factors

1.   Family predisposition
2.   Possible abnormality in dopamine neurotransmitter mechanisms of action
3.   Lower than normal levels of homovanillic acid in the cerebrospinal fluid
4.   Associated with medications

Clinical Manifestations

1.   Repetitive, sudden movements of the face, neck, or shoulders in context to normal behaviors
2.   Able to suppress movements for a period of time
3.   Involuntary movements include:
      a.   Vocal sounds (e.g., repetitive sounds)
      b.   Different movements
4.   May have learning difficulties
5.   May have obsessive behaviors
6.   Types of tics seen in children with Tourette's syndrome include:
      a.   Simple tics
          i.   Clonic
          ii.   Dystonic
      b.   Complex tics
          i.   Series of different or similar simple tics
          ii.   More complicated coordinated movements

          iii.   Copropraxia (obscene gestures) and coprographia (obscene writing)

    c.   Vocal tics

          i.   Oropharyngeal, nasopharyngeal, or laryngeal sounds

          ii.   Consonants or syllables

          iii.   Meaningful or nonsense words or phrases

          iv.   Coprolalia (obscene speech)

          v.   Palilalia (repeating one's own words) and echolalia (repeating another's words)

          vi.   Sensory tics: An indescribable, uncomfortable feeling that is relieved by a motor tic

Laboratory and/or Diagnostics

1. Metabolic screening for abnormalities:
   a. Calcium
   b. Magnesium
   c. Glucose
   d. Liver function enzymes
   e. Ceruloplasmin levels
2. Thyroid function tests
3. MRI to rule out anatomic abnormalities in the basal ganglia or metabolic abnormalities such as calcium deposition

Conditions Necessary for a Diagnosis of Tourette's Syndrome

1. Multiple motor and vocal tics variably manifested over time
2. Tics present for at least one year
3. Onset of tics before the age of 21
4. Tics not due to another known condition or substance

Differential Diagnosis

1. Simple transient tics
   a. Monomorphic tics (always the same in appearance)
   b. Last less than 12 months
   c. May be caused by particular environmental situations or psychological states
2. Chronic tics
   a. Last longer than 12 months
   b. Single type of tics

Management

1. The goals of management are to:
   a. Reduce the frequency of tics during critical circumstances with a minimum of medication side effects

      b.   Give attention to other learning or behavioral handicaps that may coexist
2.   Assess for learning disabilities and ADHD
3.   Individualized instruction/education
4.   Psychotherapy
5.   Support groups
6.   Psychological counseling for family

Pharmacotherapy

1.   Haloperidol: Doses ranging from 0.5 to 6 mg/day in divided doses
2.   Clonidine (Catapres) transdermal skin patches are very useful
3.   Pimozide (Orap): An ECG is recommended before use of this drug

Prognosis

Good for the majority of children

Sample Questions

1. Children frequently have headaches, and the most frequent chronic headache type in children is related to:

    a. Sinusitis
    b. Poor vision or eye changes
    c. Chronic daily headache or migraines
    d. Previous head injuries

2. Neurological complications of meningitis include:

    a. Mental retardation, hearing loss, and seizures
    b. Hearing loss, seizures, and severe vomiting
    c. Mental retardation, hearing loss, and glucose intolerance
    d. Decreased muscle movement, mental retardation, and hearing loss

3. Which of the following is most accurate regarding tic disorders?

    a. Tic disorders are called Tourette's syndrome
    b. Excitement, fatigue, or stress can make tics worse
    c. Tic disorders cause attention deficit hyperactivity disorder (ADHD)
    d. Medication is indicated for tics in children

Answers

1. Correct Answer: C
When a headache is present for more than 15 days per month for at least 3 months, it is described as a chronic daily headache. Often, chronic daily headaches occur every day, and some people complain that they are present continuously for months. Chronic daily headache is not a type of headache but a category that includes frequent headaches of various kinds. Most children with chronic daily headache have migraines.

2. Correct Answer: A
The neurologic complications of meningitis may be sudden or gradual in onset and can appear at any time after the onset of symptoms, including after the completion of therapy. Although many neurologic complications are severe, others, such as hearing loss, may be subtle or unapparent during the early phases of infection. The neurologic complications of meningitis include: Impaired mental status; cerebral edema and increased intracranial pressure; seizures; focal deficits (cranial nerve palsies, hemiparesis or quadriparesis). Also associated is ataxia; cerebrovascular abnormalities; neuropsychological impairment, developmental disability; subdural effusion or empyema; hydrocephalus; hypothalamic dysfunction.

3. Correct Answer: B
Not all tics are classified as Tourette's syndrome. Excitement, fatigue, and stress make all Tics worse. ADHD, obsessive-compulsive disorder, and Tourette's syndrome are all associated with each other and often occur in conjunction, but one does not cause the other. Medications are used in children if the Tics interfere with daily functioning and if other non-pharmacologic management is not successful.

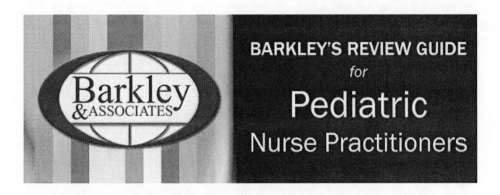

Hematological Issues and Disorders

Red Blood Cell (RBC) Indices

1.   Size: Mean corpuscular volume (MCV); expression of the average volume and size of individual erythrocytes
     a.   Microcytic: ~ < 80 fL
     b.   Normocytic: ~ 80 to 100 fL
     c.   Macrocytic: ~ 100 fL
2.   Mean corpuscular hemoglobin concentration (MCHC): Expression of the average hemoglobin (Hgb) concentration or proportion of each red blood cells (RBCs) occupied by Hbg as a percentage; "color"; more accurate measure than mean corpuscular hemoglobin (MCH)
     a.   Normochromic: 32% to 36%
     b.   Hypochromic: < 32%
     c.   Hyperchromic: > 36% (most texts deny the existence of this state, in that it is impossible for an RBC to be too red)
3.   Weight: MCH; expression of the average amount and weight of Hgb contained in a single erythrocyte; not as useful
     a.   Normal: 26 to 34 pg
4.   Red cell distribution width (RCDW)
     a.   Red cell size variation (anisocytosis)
     b.   Differentiates between iron deficiency anemia (IDA), Thalassemia, and anemia of chronic disease (ACD)
          i.   IDA: Increased
          ii.   Thalassemia: Normal or slightly increased
          iii. ACD: Normal RCDW
5.   Reticulocyte Count
     a.   Number of new, young RBCs in circulation
     b.   Expressed as a percentage (normal is 1 to 2%)
     c.   Index of bone marrow health and response to anemia
          i.   Anemia due to:
                1.   Bone marrow failure
                2.   Hemorrhage or hemolysis
          ii.   Response to therapy

Anemias

1.   Definition: Conditions caused by various disorders of the red blood cell count, quality of hemoglobin and/or volume of packed red blood cells
2.   Classification: Anemias are classified according to red blood cell size MCV
   a.   Microcytic/Hypochromic (Children): IDA, Thalassemia, lead poisoning, G6PD deficiency
   b.   Normocytic/Normochromic: ACD, acute blood loss, early IDA
   c.   Macrocytic/ Normochromic (Adult):   Vitamin B12 deficiency, folate deficiency, pernicious anemia

Microcytic Anemias

Iron Deficiency Anemia

Microcytic, hypochromatic anemia due to an overall deficiency of iron

1.   Caused by decreased iron intake, increased needs, or slow gastrointestinal (GI) blood loss
2.   In infancy, iron deficiency is due to an inadequate intake of iron (e.g., low iron formula, solely breast fed) or micro hemorrhage from the gut from early intake of whole milk (before the age of 9 months)
3.   In toddlers, iron deficiency is often due to increased reliance on whole milk at the expense of solid foods
4.   In adolescence, dieting practices contribute to inadequate intake of iron, specifically in girls after menarche

Symptoms

Severity depends on degree of anemia

1.   Easy fatigue ability
2.   Palpitations; shortness of breath on exertion
3.   Lethargy
4.   Headaches
5.   Pica
6.   Delayed motor development
7.   Pale, dry skin and mucous membranes
8.   Tachycardia
9.   Tachypnea
10.   Postural hypotension in severe anemia
11.   Brittle hair
12.   Flat, brittle or spoon shaped nails

Laboratory/Diagnostic Findings

1.   Hemoglobin and hematocrit low
2.   Low MCV

3.   Low MCHC
4.   Low RBCs
5.   Increased red cell width: Red cell distribution width (RDW)
6.   Total iron binding capacity elevated
7.   Serum ferritin < 30 ug/L
8.   Low serum iron
9.   Reticulocyte count: Low in cases of inadequate iron intake; elevated in cases of blood loss

Management

The goal of management is to correct underlying cause. A medicinal iron supplement is required while the cause is being managed and should be continued until the resolution of the underlying process

1.   Treat with elemental iron 3 to 6 mg/kg/day in one to three doses until hemoglobin (Hgb) normalizes
2.   To replace iron stores: 2 to 3 mg/kg/day for 4 months

Thalassemia

A group of hereditary disorders that are characterized by abnormal synthesis of alpha and beta globin chains

1.   Microcytosis is out of proportion to the degree of anemia

Causes/Incidence

1.   Second most common cause of microcytic anemia
2.   Autosomal, recessive genetic disorder
3.   Alpha thalassemia is more common in African Americans, Chinese, Vietnamese and Cambodians
4.   Beta thalassemia is more common in people of Mediterranean, Middle East, Indian, Southeast Asian descent

Symptoms

Depend on which chain is involved

1.   Alpha trait (one of four alpha genes affected) usually asymptomatic
2.   Alpha-thalassemia minor (two of four alpha genes affected) and Beta-thalassemia minor (heterozygous form) are mild forms, usually asymptomatic
3.   Beta-thalassemia major (Cooley's anemia with both beta genes affected): Easy fatigue ability, palpitations, shortness of breath with exertion, headaches
4.   Hemoglobin H disease (three of four alpha genes affected): Symptoms are similar to those of beta thalassemia major

Physical Exam Findings

Will usually be within normal limits, except in severe forms of thalassemia
1. Pale or bronze skin
2. Tachycardia
3. Tachypnea
4. Hepatosplenomegaly
5. Bone deformity of the face

Laboratory/Diagnostic Findings

1. General
   a. Decreased Hgb
   b. Low MCV (microcytic)
   c. Low MCHC (hypochronic)
   d. Normal total iron-binding capacity (TIBC)
   e. Normal ferritin (protein that stores iron)
   f. Decreased alpha or beta Hgb chains found on Hgb electophoresis
2. Alpha thalassemia trait
   a. Hematocrit between 28 to 40%
   b. Strikingly low MCV (60 to 75 ug/mL)
   c. Reticulocyte count normal
   d. Iron parameters normal
   e. Usually a diagnosis of exclusion in a patient with modest anemia, significant microcytosis, and no elevation of hemoglobin A2 or F
3. Alpha thalassemia minor and Beta thalassemia minor
   a. Hematocrit between 28 to 40%
   b. MCV 55 to 75 ug/mL
   c. Reticulocyte count normal or slightly elevated
   d. Iron parameters normal
   e. Hemoglobin electrophoresis shows elevation of Hgb A2 to 4 to 8% and occasional Hgb F to 1 to 5%
4. Beta thalassemia major
   a. Hematocrit may fall to < 10%
   b. MCV < 75 ug/mL
   c. Peripheral blood smear shows severe poikilocytosis, hypochromia, basophilic stippling and nucleated red blood cells
   d. Virtually no Hgb A present
   e. Major hemoglobin present is Hgb F
5. Hemoglobin H disease
   a. Hematocrit between 22 to 32%
   b. MCV < 70 ug/mL
   c. Peripheral blood smear markedly abnormal: Hypochromia, microcytosis, poikilocytosis
   d. Reticulocyte count elevated

e.   Hemoglobin electrophoresis shows Hgb H as 10 to 40% of Hgb

Management

Depends upon the type of thalassemia

1.   Patients with thalassemia trait or alpha or beta thalassemia minor are clinically normal and require no treatment; most importantly, these patients need to be evaluated and identified, so that their condition is documented and they are not subjected to repeated evaluations or inappropriately treated with iron
2.   Iron is contraindicated in all forms of thalassemia as iron overload may result
3.   Patients with Hgb H disease should take folate supplements
4.   Patients with very severe forms are maintained on a transfusion schedule
5.   If a patient's hypersplenism causes significant transfusion requirements, splenectomy is recommended
6.   Provide genetic counseling
7.   Monitor for signs/symptoms of iron overload; use deferoxamine as an iron chelating agent or to postpone hemosiderosis
8.   Allogenic bone marrow transplantation for beta thalassemia major may be needed

Sickle Cell Anemia

An anemia in which abnormal hemoglobin (due to DNA point mutation) leads to chronic hemolytic anemia and results in a variety of severe clinical consequences. The peak incidence of infection is between ages 1 and 3

Causes/Incidence

1.   Autosomal recessive disorder in which Hgb S develops instead of Hgb A. The patient is homozygous for Hgb S (Hgb SS)
2.   Most prevalent in persons of African or African American ancestry; Hgb S gene is carried in 8% of African Americans : Incidence is 1 to 400
3.   Patients who have heterozygous genotype (Hgb AS) are generally clinically normal but are carriers

Symptoms

1.   Sickle Cell Trait (Hgb AS)
        a.   Patients usually have no clinical symptoms
        b.   May experience acute painful symptoms under extreme conditions such as exertion at high altitudes
2.   Sickle Cell Anemia (Hgb SS)
        a.   Sudden, excruciating pain due to a vaso-occlusive crisis usually in the back, chest, abdomen and long bones
        b.   Low grade fever

235

c.   Predisposing factors may be present (e.g., infection, physical or emotional stress, blood loss)

<u>Physical Exam Findings</u>

1.   Sickle Cell Trait
   a.   These patients are clinically normal with no abnormal exam findings
2.   Sickle Cell Anemia
   a.   Chronically ill in appearance
   b.   Jaundice
   c.   Retinopathy
   d.   Delayed puberty
   e.   Hepatosplenomegaly
   f.   Spleen usually not palpable in the adult
   g.   Enlarged heart with hyperdynamic precordium
   h.   Systolic murmur
   i.   Non-healing ulcers of the lower leg may be present
   j.   Fatigue
   k.   Tendency toward more frequent infections (which also aggravates crisis)

<u>Laboratory/Diagnostic Findings</u>

1.   Hematocrit 20 to 30%
2.   Irreversibly sickled cells on peripheral blood smear (5 to 50% of total)
3.   Reticulocytosis (10 to 25%)
4.   Nucleated red blood cells
5.   Howell-Jolly bodies and target cells
6.   White blood cells (WBC) characteristically elevated to 12,000 to 15,000
7.   Indirect bilirubin elevated
8.   Platelets may be elevated (> 400,000)
9.   Sickledex test is used for screening; sickle cells are present in patients with trait and anemia
10.   Hemoglobin electrophoresis shows 85 to 95% Hgb S in sickle cell anemia and approximately 40% Hgb S in sickle cell trait
11.   Hemoglobin F may be present
12.   Children with sickle cell trait may have episodes of gross hematuria and inability to concentrate the urine due to renal tubular defect

<u>Management</u>

1.   No specific treatment; mainly palliative or symptomatic relief
2.   Maintained chronically on folic acid supplementation
3.   Cornerstone of therapy is support during crisis
   a.   Keep client well hydrated
   b.   Ensure adequate oxygenation

c. Analgesics for pain control
d. Antibiotics for associated infection
e. Exchange transfusions for treatment of intractable crisis as a preventative measure for clients undergoing anesthesia
4. Hydroxyurea 500 to 750 mg/daily when quality of life interrupted by frequent crises
5. Provide or refer for genetic counseling

Lead Poisoning

Chronic disease as the result of toxic accumulation of lead in the body. The Centers for Disease Control and Prevention (CDC) definition of lead poisoning is a level > 19 ug/dL; can occur via ingestion or inhalation. Highest prevalence among poor, inner-city children and those living in old housing

Common Sources

1. Paint and paint dust
2. Contaminated soil
3. Gasoline emissions
4. Food and drinking water
5. Mexican-American, Asian, Indian, or other ethnic folk remedies

Signs/Symptoms

1. Vague: GI symptoms
2. Severe: Lethargy, difficult walking, neuropathies
3. Headaches
4. Burtonian lines: Bluish discoloration of gingival border
5. Ataxia
6. Papilledema

Laboratory/Diagnostics

1. Class I: Level < 10 ug/dL
2. Class IIA: Level 10 to 14 ug/dL
3. Class IIB: Level 15 to 19 ug/dL
4. Class III: Level 20 to 24 ug/dL
5. Class IV: Level 25 to 69 ug/dL
6. Class V: Level > 70 ug/dL
7. May cause hemoglobinopathies
8. Impaired renal function, vitamin D metabolism

Management

1. Class I: None
2. Class II: Screen every 3 to 4 months; provide education
3. Classes III, IV and V: Further evaluation

  a. Iron deficiency
  b. Environmental assessment
4. Classes IV and V require chelation

Glucose-6-Phosphate Dehydrogenase Deficiency (G6PD)

Autosomal recessive disorder in which the enzyme is decreased or absent:
Exacerbations may be caused by certain drugs and foods; most common in
Mediterranean and African American persons

Drugs and Foods to Avoid

1. Aspirin (ASA)
2. Sulfonamides
3. Antimalarials
4. Fava beans
5. Exposure to pollen from the bean's flower

Signs/Symptoms

1. Weakness
2. Pallor
3. Splenomegaly
4. Neonatal jaundice
5. Jaundice during acute episodes

Laboratory/Diagnostics

1. Flourescence based screen
2. Red blood cell indices after episode
  a. Heinz bodies
  b. Blister cells
3. Reticulocytosis

Management

1. Avoid triggering foods/drugs
2. Transfusion for severe crisis

Leukemias

A group of malignant hematological diseases in which normal bone marrow
elements are replaced by abnormal, poorly differentiated lymphocytes known as
blast cells

1. Acute lymphocytic leukemia (ALL) accounts for about 75% of cases, a peak
    incidence around 4 years of age. It occurs more frequently in boys than
    girls and is more common among African Americans than Caucasians

2.   Acute myelogenous leukemia (AML) accounts for about 20% of all leukemias and occurs primarily in older children
3.   Chronic myelogenous leukemia (CML) is an adult form of the disease seen in < 3% of children. The exact cause of this disease is unknown, however, factors such as infection, radiation, chemical and drug exposure and genetic factors are associated risk

Signs/Symptoms

1.   Anemia
2.   Pale
3.   Listless
4.   Irritable
5.   Chronically tired
6.   History of repeated infections
7.   Bleeding such as epistaxis, petechiae, and hematomas
8.   Lymphadenopathy and hepatosplenomegaly
9.   Bone and joint pain

Laboratory/Diagnostics

1.   Complete blood count (CBC) with differential WBC, platelet and reticulocyte counts (thrombocytopenia is present in up to 85% of cases, and anemia is usually present)
2.   Peripheral smear may demonstrate malignant cells
3.   Bone marrow will show blast cells replacing normal elements

Management

1.   Referral to an oncologist
2.   Supportive care of family
3.   Provide information on support groups and other community resources

Sample Questions

1. A 24-month-old African-American female presents to the clinic with complaints from her parents of being "unusually tired." She has no history of chronic illness. The history reveals that she was switched to whole milk at 12 months of age and is currently drinking 32 oz. per day. Upon examination, you notice pale conjunctiva, and laboratory results reveal microcytic hypochromic anemia with normal white blood cell (WBC) count, platelet count, and reticulocyte count. What diagnosis is most likely at this point?

    a. Sickle cell anemia
    b. Alpha-thalassemia minor
    c. Iron deficiency anemia (IDA)
    d. Vitamin B-12 deficiency

2. Which of the following patients would you most likely suspect to be in need of a transfusion?

    a. A sickle cell disease patient with a pain crisis
    b. A beta-thalassemia major patient with shortness of breath
    c. A child with newly-diagnosed IDA
    d. A child with class III lead poisoning

3. You are evaluating an infant who had prenatal exposure to lead. Which of the following would be the most likely symptom?

    a. Abdominal pain
    b. Vomiting
    c. Slowed growth
    d. Muscle weakness

Answers

1. Correct Answer: C

Sickle cell anemia would most likely also have icteric sclera, elevated white blood cells, and reticulocytosis. Sickle cell disease is one of the mandatory newborn screening tests for all states in the nation and should be picked up in infancy. Although the child is African-American, nothing else fits to make sickle cell disease a good choice. Alpha thalassemia minor is usually asymptomatic. Vitamin B12 deficiency is macrocytic and normochromic, and meat or dairy products such as milk are a good source. Iron deficiency anemia is the correct answer. It is sometimes difficult to assess pale skinned African-Americans, but looking at the conjunctiva, which is normally pink, is a good way to assess for this. In infancy, increased whole milk or whole milk too early can lead to gastrointestinal blood loss and iron deficiency anemia. In toddlers, IDA is caused by the increased reliance on whole milk at the expense of whole foods.

2. Correct Answer: B

Sickle cell disease patients require blood transfusions for acute chest syndrome, stroke, and severe symptoms of anemia but not always for pain crisis. Beta-thalassemia patients are in need of chronic transfusions, especially when they are symptomatic. A child with newly diagnosed IDA will most likely require iron to return the hemogobin back to normal. Class III lead poisoning requires further evaluation but no transfusion.

3. Correct Answer: C

Abdominal pain and vomiting are seen in children who have been exposed to lead. Muscle weakness is seen in adults with lead exposure. Infants exposed in utero will most likely have slowed growth and learning difficulties.

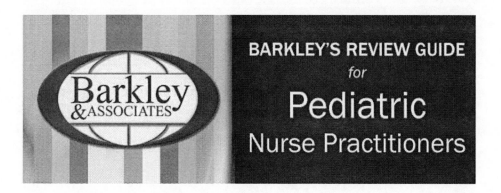

BARKLEY'S REVIEW GUIDE
for
Pediatric
Nurse Practitioners

Endocrine Issues and Disorders

Diabetes Mellitus

Represents a syndrome with disordered metabolism and inappropriate hyperglycemia due to either an absolute deficiency of insulin secretion or a reduction in its biologic effectiveness

1. Age of onset is not a criterion
2. Diabetes mellitus (DM) is classified as either type 1 or type 2
3. Type 1 produces ketosis in the untreated state, and type 2 usually does not

Type 1 Diabetes Mellitus

1. Previously known as insulin-dependent or juvenile diabetes
2. Most common in juveniles
3. Certain human leukocyte antigens are strongly associated with the development
   a. 85 to 95% of patients have serotype HLA-DR3 or HLA-DR4
4. Circulating islet cell antibodies can be detected in the first few weeks after presentation in 85% of patients
5. Believed to be the result of an infectious or toxic environmental insult to pancreatic B cells of genetically predisposed persons

Signs/Symptoms

1. Polyuria, polydipsia, and polyphagia are classic
2. Nocturnal enuresis
3. Weight loss, with increased hunger
4. Fatigue, weakness, paraesthesia
5. If onset is very acute, may have level of consciousness (LOC) changes ranging from irritability to coma
6. Loss of subcutaneous (SQ) fat and muscle wasting suggestive of insidious onset
7. Dysfunction of peripheral sensory nerves
8. Skin and vaginal infections
9. In advanced disease:

      a.   Ophthalmic exam may reveal microaneurysms or cotton wool spots

      b.   Evidence of peripheral vascular insufficiency

      c.   Diminished deep tendon reflexes (DTRs)

10.   May show evidence of dehydration

Differential Diagnosis

1.   Type 2 DM
2.   Pancreatitis
3.   Secondary effects of drug therapy

Laboratory/Diagnostics

1.   Serum fasting blood sugar $\geq$ 126 mg/dL on two separate occasions is diagnostic
2.   Random blood sugar $\geq$ 200 mg/dL and polydipsia, polyuria and weight loss indicate the need to confirm the diagnosis by fasting studies
3.   Glucosuria
4.   Ketonuria
5.   Plasma ketones
6.   Serum blood urea nitrogen (BUN) and creatinine may be elevated
7.   Hemoglobin (Hgb) A_{1c} (normal: 5.5 to 7%)
8.   Impaired glucose tolerance: Fasting blood glucose (FBG) $\geq$ 100 and $\leq$ 125

Distinguishing Type 1 from Type 2: Laboratory/Diagnostics

1.   Increased plasma levels
2.   Markers of autoimmune B-cell destruction

Management

1.   Need to establish baseline studies

      a.   Family history

      b.   Age of onset of DM, presence of obesity, whether insulin required

      c.   Note presence of cardiac risk factors

      d.   Note diagnostic markers

      e.   Note presence or absence of ketones

      f.   Baseline fasting triglycerides, cholesterol, renal studies, electrocardiogram (ECG)

      g.   Baseline physical exam including peripheral pulses, neuro exam, foot exam

2.   Dietary teaching: May consult dietitian

      a.   Total carbohydrate intake: 50 to 60% of total caloric intake

      b.   Fats: 25 to 30% of total calories

      c.   Fiber: 25g/1,000 calories

      d.   Cholesterol: 300 mg/day

      e.   Protein: 10 to 20% of total calories

    f.   Total caloric intake to achieve ideal body weight
3.   Patients presenting with ketones must start insulin; the rule of thumb is to begin with 0.5 u/kg/day, giving 2/3 of the dose in the morning and the remaining 1/3 in the evening

Conventional split dose insulin

1.   The morning dose is 2/3 neutral protamine Hagedorn (NPH) insulin and 1/3 regular human insulin (R)
2.   The evening dose is 1/2 NPH and 1/2 R
3.   A 70 kg patient would get 35 units of insulin daily
    a.   10 units of R and 15 units of NPH in the morning
    b.   5 units of R and 5 units of NPH in the evening

Intensive Insulin Therapy

1.   Reduce or omit the evening dose and add a portion at bedtime (HS for "hour of sleep")
    a.   5 units of R in the evening
    b.   5 units of NPH at HS

Alternatives

1.   Alternative #1
    a.   3 daily doses of short- or ultra-short-acting insulin prior to meals
    b.   Based on carbohydrate counting
    c.   1 unit of insulin per 10 to 15 grams of carbs
    d.   1 dose of long acting insulin (ultralente) pre-breakfast and pre-dinner
    e.   Dose is 0.5 × weight in kg/2, split equally
2.   Alternative #2
    a.   3 daily shots of short- or ultra-short-acting insulin prior to meals
    b.   Based on carbohydrate units
    c.   Single dose of insulin (Lantus) at HS
    d.   0.5 × weight in kg/2
3.   Alternative #3
    a.   Combines short or ultra-short and intermediate acting (NPH) insulin
    b.   Pre-meal: Short- or ultra-short-acting based on carbohydrate units
    c.   NPH total daily dose = 0.5 × weight in kg/2
    d.   Half of NPH given in the evening
    e.   Remaining NPH divided evenly among the 3 meals and administered with short- or ultra-short-acting insulin

Somogyi Effect and the Dawn Phenomenon

Two conditions that result in early morning hyperglycemia but have different etiologies and different management strategies

1.   The Somogyi effect results when nocturnal hypoglycemia stimulates a surge of counter regulatory hormones that raise blood sugar; this patient is hypoglycemic at 3 a.m., and rebounds with an elevated blood sugar at 7 a.m.
      a.   Treatment: Reduce or eliminate the HS dose of insulin
2.   The Dawn Phenomenon results when tissue becomes desensitized to insulin nocturnally; blood sugar gets progressively higher throughout the night, and is elevated at 7 a.m.; this desensitization is felt to be due to the presence of growth hormone, which spikes at night
      a.   Treatment: Add or increase the dose of HS insulin

Type 2 Diabetes Mellitus

1.   Previously referred to as non-insulin-dependent diabetes mellitus [(non-IDDM) or adult onset DM]
2.   90% diabetics in the U.S. are of this type
3.   Not linked to human leukocyte antigen system (HLA)
4.   No islet cell antibodies
5.   Presence of obesity or family history increases risk

Signs/Symptoms

1.   Insidious onset of hyperglycemia may be asymptomatic
2.   Generalized pruritus
3.   Recurrent vaginitis is often the first symptom in women
4.   Peripheral neuropathies and recurrent blurred vision are more common than in type 1
5.   Chronic skin infections
6.   Acanthosis nigricans
7.   Polydipsia, polyphagia, polyuria less common symptoms for type 2 DM
8.   In early disease, physical findings are unremarkable
9.   In advanced disease, physical findings are similar to type 1 DM

Differential Diagnosis

1.   Type 1 DM
2.   Other endocrine disorders resulting in carbohydrate intolerance
3.   Secondary effects of medication
4.   Pancreatitis
5.   Liver disease

Laboratory/Diagnostics

1.   Screening: Fasting blood glucose levels
2.   Same as for type 1 DM except for the presence of ketones in blood/urine

Consider screening if:

1. The patient is overweight [body mass index (BMI) > 85% for age and gender] and has 2 of the following risk factors:
    a. Family history of type 2 DM in first or second-degree relative
    b. Race/ethnicity of African American, Native American, Hispanic, or Asian/Pacific Islanders
    c. Signs associated with insulin resistance:
        i. Acanthosis nigricans
        ii. Hypertension
        iii. Dyslipidemia
        iv. Polycystic ovarian disease
2. Screening, if done, should begin at age 10 or onset of puberty (whichever occurs first); repeat every 2 years

Management

1. Obtain baseline data as outlined for type 1 DM
2. Therapy should begin with weight control for obese clients
3. Initial therapy consists of dietary treatment with dietary guidelines as outlined in the management of type 1 DM
4. If dietary management is unsuccessful, begin treatment with oral antidiabetics
5. Need to institute insulin therapy in addition to oral therapy for patients who present with hyperglycemia with diabetic ketoacidosis (DKA); eventually, the insulin is discontinued

Oral Antidiabetics

1. Five most common classes of oral agents [only one of these drugs, metformin (Glucophage), is currently FDA-approved for use in children]
2. Sulfonylureas, alpha-glucosidase inhibitors, Non-sulfonylurea insulin release stimulators and Glucovance are not approved for use in children

Biguanides

1. Metformin (850 mg twice a day or 500 mg three times a day)
    a. Does not stimulate insulin action, but it reduces gluconeogenesis
    b. Not metabolized: Is excreted unchanged
    c. Good adjunct to sulfonylureas but can be used alone: Especially for the obese
    d. Should not be given in hepatic or renal failure, alcoholics, or those prone to hypoxia
    e. Significant gastrointestinal upset
    f. Little or no hypoglycemia
    g. Need to be discharged 48 hours before a procedure

Hyperthyroidism

Hyperthyroidism or thyrotoxicosis denotes a series of clinical disorders associated with increased circulating levels of free thyroxine or triiodothyronine

1.   Grave's disease is the most common and is associated with diffuse enlargement of thyroid, hyperactivity of the gland, and the presence of antibodies against different fractions of the thyroid gland

Causes/Incidence

1.   More common in females (8:1)
2.   Onset between 12 and 14 years of age
3.   Other causes of hyperthyroidism include toxic adenoma, subacute thyroiditis, thyroid-stimulating hormone (TSH)-secreting pituitary tumor, and high dose amiodarone

Signs/Symptoms

1.   Nervousness
2.   Restlessness
3.   Increased sweating
4.   Muscle cramps
5.   Frequent basilar migraine
6.   Weight changes (usually a loss)
7.   Palpitations
8.   Angina pectoris
9.   Menstrual irregularities
10.   Warm moist skin
11.   Fine hair
12.   Heat intolerance

Other Physical Findings

1.   Atrial fibrillation
2.   Tachycardia
3.   Resting tremors
4.   Warm, moist skin
5.   Thyroid goiter (often without bruit)
6.   Grave's ophthalmopathy may be present
7.   Thin muscle wasting
8.   Hyperactive deep tendon reflexes (DTRs)

Laboratory/Diagnostics

1.   Serum thyroxine T3, triiodothyronine T4, thyroid resin uptake, and free thyroxine index increased
2.   Sometimes free T4 is high normal and can be increased, T4 is elevated, and T3 elevated (80 to 230 ng/dL)

3.   Reliable TSH assay is the most sensitive test; will show suppression except in rare cases (normal 0.5 to 5.0 uU/ml)
4.   Serum antinuclear antibodies (ANA) usually elevated without evidence of lupus or other collagen disease

Management

1.   Propranolol for symptomatic relief: Begin dosing with 10 mg, may go to 80 mg four times daily
2.   Thiourea drugs for patients with mild cases, small goiters or fear of isotopes
    a.   High rate of recurrent hyperthyroidism after 1 year of therapy
    b.   Methimazole 30 to 60 mg once daily
    c.   Propylthiouracil 300 to 600 mg daily in 4 divided doses
3.   Radioactive iodine 131-I
4.   Thyroid surgery (must be euthyroid preoperatively)
5.   Two to 3 drops of Lugol's solution every day × 10 days to reduce the vascularity of the gland

Hypothyroidism

A condition resulting in lack of circulating thyroid hormone

1.   May be due to disease of the thyroid gland itself or to a deficiency of pituitary thyroid-stimulating hormone (TSH) or hypothalamic thyrotropin-releasing hormone (TRH)
2.   Most often due to autoimmune thyroiditis, other causes include iodine deficiency, deficient pituitary, and destruction of the gland by surgery or external radiation

Causes/Incidence

1.   Congenital
    a.   May affect fetus in first trimester
    b.   Absence or underdevelopment of the thyroid gland
    c.   Inherent dysfunction in transport/assimilation of iodine
    d.   Hypothalmic or pituitary disorder
    e.   Occurs in 1:4,000 live births
2.   Juvenile acquired
    a.   Hashimoto's thyroiditis
    b.   Pituitary deficiency of TSH
    c.   Hypothalamic deficiency of TRH
    d.   Iodide deficiency
    e.   Damage to the gland

Signs/Symptoms: Neonates/Infants

1.   No obvious symptoms in the first month of life

2.   Lethargy, poor feeding, prolonged bilirubin elevation
3.   Growth deceleration
4.   Large fontanels
5.   Bradycardia
6.   Hypotonia

Signs/Symptoms: Older Children

1.   Weakness, muscle fatigue
2.   Poor growth
3.   Arthralgias
4.   Cramps
5.   Cold intolerance
6.   Constipation
7.   Weight gain
8.   Mental/physical sluggishness
9.   Poor motor coordination
10.   Delayed bone age
11.   Dry skin
12.   Thinning hair
13.   Brittle nails
14.   Puffy eyes
15.   Thick tongue
16.   Edema of the hands and face
17.   Alopecia
18.   Slowed deep tendon reflexes (DTRs)
19.   Ascites
20.   Hypoactive bowel sounds
21.   Diminished heart sounds

Laboratory/Diagnostic Findings

1.   Newborn is screening mandatory in all states
2.   Elevated TSH
3.   T4 and free T4 are both low or low normal
4.   Increased serum cholesterol
5.   Increased liver enzymes
6.   Hyponatremia, hypoglycemia
7.   Anemia
8.   Serum T3 is not a good test for hypothyroidism

Management

1.   Refer to a pediatric endocrinologist
2.   Hormone replacement therapy with levothyroxine is drug of choice

Short Stature

1.   Height falling > 2 standard deviations (SD) below mean, or a marked deviation from previously established growth curve
2.   Failure to grow more than 4 cm per year
3.   5% of the population

Growth

1.   Target height range is calculated as mid-parental stature ± 2 SD (1 SD to 2 inches)
2.   Mid-parental stature for boys is (paternal height + maternal height + 5 inches)/2
3.   Mid-parental stature for girls is (paternal height + maternal height to 5 inches)/2

Normal Variants

1.   Familial genetic variant
      a.   Normal linear growth velocity and a short target height
2.   Constitutional delay: Bone age consistent with height age
      a.   Slow growth rate for the first 2 to 3 years of life, then a low-normal growth velocity
      b.   Family history of short stature and delayed puberty are often present

Proportional Short Stature

1.   Intrauterine growth restriction (IUGR)
2.   Maternal/fetal infection
3.   Chromosomal abnormalities
4.   Failure to thrive
5.   Variety of endocrine diseases
      a.   Hypopituitarism
      b.   Growth hormone (GH) deficiency
      c.   Diabetes
      d.   Hypothyroidism

Disproportionate Stature

1.   Dwarfism
2.   Rickets

Signs/Symptoms

1.   Assess for chronic disease, neglect, endocrine deficiencies
2.   Investigate underlying causes based upon proportion

Laboratory/Diagnostics

1. CBC, liver function tests (LFTs), electrolytes, erythrocyte sedimentation rate (ESR)
2. Bone age (consider skeletal survey for disproportionate features)
3. Urinalysis including pH and specific gravity
4. Thyroid function test
5. Antiendomysial and antigliadin antibodies for celiac disease
6. Stool for ova and parasites (O and P)
7. Growth hormone
8. Sweat test if recurrent bronchitis

Management

1. Depends upon cause
2. Refer to endocrinology as appropriate
3. Family support
4. Growth hormone injections when indicated

Sample Questions

1. The mother of a 6-year-old diabetic reports that her child's blood sugar in the middle of the night during sleep was 59 mg/dL, but was 210 at 7am when she awoke. What would you most likely recommend with regard to the insulin regimen?

    a. Inform the mother that this is not likely and get her to recheck the following evening
    b. Eliminate the insulin given at bedtime
    c. Inform the parent that this is called the "Dawn Phenomenon" and increase the insulin given at bedtime
    d. Change the bedtime insulin to long regular

2. You are taking a history from a 15-year-old who complains of being tired all the time; has dry, flaky skin and puffiness around the eyes, and depression. You will do a thorough examination and order some lab work, including what?

    a. CBC, Electrolytes, BUN
    b. TSH, T4
    c. T3 and Thyroxin test
    d. Urine for Thyroxin, T3, T4

3. A diagnosis of short stature should be considered in any child failing to grow at least how many centimeters per year?

    a. 2 cm
    b. 3 cm
    c. 4 cm
    d. 5 cm

Answers

1. Correct Answer: B

This is most likely the Somogyi effect where nocturnal hypoglycemia stimulates a surge of counter regulatory hormones that raise blood sugar; this results in a hypoglycemic patient at 3am and a hyperglycemic patient at 7am; the treatment for this is to reduce or eliminate the bedtime insulin. The Dawn Phenomenon results when tissue become desensitized to insulin nocturnally and blood sugar gets progressively higher throughout the night and is elevated at 7am. Changing the bedtime insulin to regular would result in more pronounce hypoglycemia at 3 am or earlier since it peaks in 2 to 4 hours, and it has a 4 to 6 hour duration.

2. Correct Answer: B

When hypothyroidism develops in older children before growth and development are complete, they may have a shorter-than-average height or puberty may be delayed. They also may have symptoms that are more like those found in adults: Slow heart rate; tiredness; inability to tolerate cold; dry, flaky skin; puffiness in the face, especially around the eyes; impaired memory and difficulty thinking (which may appear as a new learning disability); depression; drowsiness, despite sleeping through the night; heavy or irregular menstrual periods (in girls at the age of puberty); constipation.

3. Correct Answer: C

Short stature, which is present in 5% of the population, is indicated by a failure to grow more than 4 cm per year, height falling > 2 standard deviations (SD) below mean, or a marked deviation from previously established growth curve.

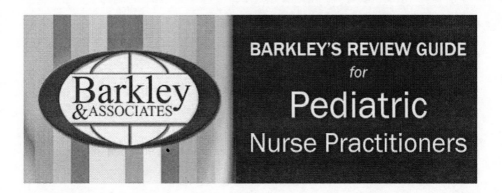

BARKLEY'S REVIEW GUIDE
for
Pediatric
Nurse Practitioners

Genitourinary and Gynecological Issues and Disorders

Enuresis

Involuntary urination occurs at an age when voluntary control should be present.

Types noted as follows:

1. Primary enuresis: Children who have never established control
2. Secondary enuresis: Present when children have been dry for more than 6 to 12 months and begin wetting
3. Nocturnal enuresis: Incontinence during sleep
4. Diurnal enuresis: Occurs during waking hours

Incidence

The incidence of enuresis is difficult to assess; however, the estimated rates are:

1. 40% in 3-year-olds
2. 7 to 10% in 5-year-olds
3. 2 to 3% in 10-year-olds
4. More boys are affected with nocturnal enuresis
5. A greater number of African-American children are affected when compared to Caucasian children
6. Approximately 95% of cases are functional

Signs/Symptoms

1. History of bed wetting
2. A diurnal enuresis history of immediate urgency, restless or jiggly leg crossing, and/or holding private areas

Laboratory/Diagnostics

1. Urinalysis (UA)
2. Urine culture

Management

1. Functional enuresis
   a. Enuresis alarm

      b.   Positive reinforcement such as utilizing a star chart

      c.   Bladder control training (geared toward training the bladder to hold more urine)

      d.   Pharmacological therapy:

          i.   Imipramine 25 mg daily 1 hour before bedtime × 1 week, increase to 50 mg for children ages 6 to 12years, 75 mg for children older than 12 years

          ii.   Desmopressin (DDAVP):

              1.   Orally: 0.2 mg tablets once daily at bedtime (HS for "hour of sleep"), can adjust up to maximum of 0.6 mg/dose

              2.   Nasal spray or solution: 20 ug (2 sprays) or 0.2 ml solution intranasally at bedtime; can adjust upward to 40 ug or down to 10 ug/dose

          iii.   Oxybutynin (Ditropan): If less than 6 years for detrusor muscle hyperactivity associated with neurological disorders (spina bifida); 5 mg may be given twice a day to a maximum of 5 mg three times daily

              Note: Children using drug therapy should have a drug holiday every 3 months to assess the need for continued pharmacotherapy; after 1 month without wetting, medication can be tapered over a 2-to-4-week period; there is a high rate of relapse when medication is discontinued; however, it is useful for overnight outings

      e.   Hypnosis and self-hypnosis (better success rate than medication use)

      f.   Parent education

2.   Organic causes: Treat the underlying cause [the most common is a urinary tract infection (UTI)]

Urinary Tract Infection

Bacterial infections and inflammation of the urinary tract are more common in males (uncircumcised) in the first year of life; increases are seen in females (short urethra of 3 to 4 cm) at a 10:1 ratio throughout the lifespan.

1.   Both male and female UTIs in childhood are typically caused by the following organisms:

      a.   *E. Coli*: 80 to 90% of uncomplicated UTIs; 20% of complicated UTIs

      b.   *Staphyloccoccus aureus*: Majority of complicated UTIs

2.   Common predisposing factors include urinary stasis, congenital or acquired obstructive lesions, non-obstructive causes (e.g., neurogenic bladder, poor hygiene, constipation, and sexual intercourse)

3.   In 25 to 50% of children, a repeat UTI may occur, especially during the first year following the initial UTI
4.   Newborn and young infants with UTIs, especially those with high-grade vesicoureteral reflex (VUR), may potentially experience renal scarring, eventual hypertension, and renal failure
5.   Types of UTIs:
    a.   Uncomplicated UTIs: Cystitis or pyelonephritis that develop in absence of structural abnormality, obstruction, or other disease
    b.   Complicated UTIs: Chronic cystitis or pyelonephritis that develop in the presence of structural abnormality, obstruction, or other disease

Signs/Symptoms

1.   In infants:
    a.   Weight loss
    b.   Failure to thrive
    c.   Dehydration
    d.   Irritability
2.   May be no appreciable signs and symptoms
3.   Classic findings that may be present in adolescents:
    a.   Dysuria
    b.   Frequency
    c.   Nocturia
    d.   Urgency
    e.   Suprapubic/lower abdominal discomfort
    f.   Hematuria
    g.   Fever

Laboratory/Diagnostics

1.   A straight catheter (cath) is indicated in those who cannot void voluntarily
2.   Clean catch may be used for mild symptoms or follow-up
3.   Gram stain and culture of organisms.
4.   UA: Leukocytes, erythrocytes, nitrites
5.   Leukocytosis in the complete blood count (CBC)
6.   Girls less than 5 years old and boys of any age who are febrile should have renal ultrasonography and voiding cystourethrogram (VCUG) after the first UTI

Management

1.   Simple UTI: Antibiotic therapy for 3 to 10 days
2.   Children less than 2 months of age:
    a.   Bactrim DS
    b.   Cephalosporins
    c.   Amoxicillin

      d.   Sulfisoxazole

      e.   Nitrofurantoin

           Note: Children < 2 months of age diagnosed with a UTI should be hospitalized and receive parenteral antibiotics

3. Encourage fluids; cranberry juice, although not proven, is believed to prevent bacteria from adhering to uroepithelial cells
4. Frequent bladder emptying
5. Proper wiping
6. Follow-up in 2 days; change antibiotic if no improvement is seen
7. Follow-up in 1 to 2 weeks, then every 1 to 3 months for 1 year
8. For those with VUR: Low-dose antibiotics (Bactrim) for 1 year following treatment for acute infection
9. Males (6 to 15 years) with first infection: Refer to urologist for full evaluation

Glomerulonephritis (GN)

A non-infectious, inflammatory response of the kidney glomeruli (in the primary form of the disease), characterized by varied degrees of hypertension, edema, proteinuria, and hematuria

1. Secondary glomerulonephritis occurs when renal involvement is secondary to systemic disease (e.g., lupus, primary vasculitis, drug hypersensitivity reactions)
2. Poststreptococcal glomerulonephritis (PSGN) is the classic form of GN and is the most common form of nephritis in childhood
3. Occurs more often in males (2:1); peaks at 7 years of age
4. Is unusual in children less than 3 years of age

Signs/Symptoms

1. History of streptococcal infection
2. Abrupt onset of gross hematuria
3. Reduced urine output
4. Lethargy, anorexia, nausea, vomiting, abdominal or flank pain
5. Chills, fever, back pain
6. Hypertension
7. Periorbiatal edema
8. Oliguria
9. May have a rash or arthralgias (secondary to lupus, impetigo)
10. Trauma or abuse

Laboratory/Diagnostics

1. UA with microscopic tea color urine, elevated specific gravity, macro and microhematuria, proteinuria, pyuria with acute poststreptococcal

glomerulonephris (PSGN), granular, hyaline, white blood cells (WBC) or red blood cells (RBC), and dysmorphic RBCs

2.   Serum C3/C4: Low in the early phase of disease; back to normal within 6 to 8 weeks
3.   CBC, erythrocyte sedimentation rate (ESR), antistreptolysin O (ASO) titer (elevated), Streptozyme test (positive), anti-DNase-B titer
4.   Electrolytes, blood urea nitrogen (BUN), creatinine, and cholesterol
5.   Hepatitis titer, sickle cell or hemoglobin electrophoresis, tuberculin purified protein derivative (PPD), and fluorescent treponemal antibody absorption (syphilis), should be ordered as appropriate

Management

1.   Referral to a nephrologist for post streptococcal glomerular nephritis (PSGN) supportive care
2.   Hospitalization in the acute phase
3.   Follow-up treatment requires monitoring of blood pressure (BP), UA and renal function annually

Hypospadias

A relatively common congenital abnormality in which the urethral opening is on the ventral surface (underside) of the penis

1.   The etiology is unclear; currently hypothesized to be a deformity rather than a malformation
2.   Occurs in 8.2:1,000 live births or 1:300 male infants
3.   If there is a family history of hypospadias, the risk increases in offspring
4.   Likelihood of other genitourinary (GU) anomalies such as undescended testicles, inguinal hernia, or hydrocele is noted

Sign/Symptoms

1.   Sits to void or holds penis to direct stream
2.   Dorsally hooded foreskin (classic finding)
3.   Urinary stream that aims downward
4.   Chordee (ventral bowing of the penis)
5.   Urethral opening (classification made by location):
       a.   Anterior (70%): Glandular, coronal, or anterior penile
       b.   Middle (10%)
       c.   Posterior (20%): Scrotal, penoscrotal, or posterior penile

Laboratory/Diagnostics

1.   No lab tests
2.   Diagnosis is made by clinical findings

Management

1.   Referral to a urologist at birth
2.   Circumcision must not be done (foreskin is used in repair)
3.   Surgery best done around 6 to 12 months of age

Cryptorchidism (Undescended Testes)

Absence of one or both of the testes from the scrotal sac due to failure to descend from abdomen in utero

1.   Occurs in 3% of newborn males and 20 to 30% of premature male newborns (descent normally occurs during the last trimester)

Signs/Symptoms

1.   Inability to palpate testicle
2.   Often no symptoms

Laboratory/Diagnostics

1.   None typically
2.   If bilateral, karyotyping for chromosomal abnormalities may be ordered

Management

1.   If undescended by one year, refer to urology
2.   Testicular self-examination (TSE) for testicular cancer probability

Testicular Torsion

Twisting and strangulation of the spermatic cord, characterized by acute pain; constitutes a surgical emergency to prevent necrotic testicle and infertility

Causes/Incidence

1.   Occurs most often in the 10 to 20 age group
2.   Does not represent an infectious process
3.   Interruption of the vascular flow produces acute pain

Signs/Symptoms

1.   Acute onset creates profound pain
2.   Lack of irritative voiding symptoms
3.   No systemic symptoms and no fever
4.   The affected testis may have a "high lie"
5.   Pain is not relieved by elevating scrotum

Laboratory/Diagnostics

1.   None in primary care

Management

1.   Refer for emergent surgical intervention

Dysmenorrhea

Pain and cramping associated with menstraution

1.   Primary:
   a.   Absence of any pelvic pathology; is most commonly seen in adolescents
   b.   The etiology of primary dysmenorrhea is believed to be hormonal and endocrine-related
   c.   Most cases of primary dysmenorrhea begin 6 to 12 months after menarche, with symptoms gradually increasing until patients are in their mid-20s
2.   Secondary dysmenorrhea results from an underlying cause such as pregnancy, pelvic inflammatory disease (PID), and endometriosis

Signs/Symptoms

1.   Painful menses
2.   Lower abdominal pain associated with menstruation, usually worse in the first few days of bleeding
3.   Associated back pain
4.   May have nausea, vomiting, fatigue, headache, and diarrhea

Laboratory/Diagnostics

1.   Primary dysmenorrhea: No testing as necessary diagnosis is made clinically
2.   Testing for secondary dysmenorrhea: According to suspected underlying cause

Management

1.   Education about menstruation, proper diet
2.   Support measures:
   a.   Heat application
   b.   Psychological support
   c.   Over the counter (OTC) analgesics, preferably ibuprofen: 400 mg every 4 to 6 hours, beginning at the onset of menstrual cycle and continuing for 24 to 72 hours
3.   Stronger non-steroidal anti-inflammatory drugs (NSAID) for moderate to severe dysmenorrhea
4.   Oral contraceptives
5.   Referral as needed

Sexually-Transmitted Diseases and Infections

The majority of teenagers in the United States have their first sexual experiences before graduating from high school. The consequences include increased rates of bacterial and viral sexually-transmitted diseases/infections (STDs/STIs), unintended pregnancy, and the emergence of acquired immunodeficiency syndrome (AIDS) as the 6th leading cause of death in the 15 to 24 year age group. It has been estimated that about 4% of high school students have at least one STD/STI.

Chlamydia

A parasitic sexually-transmitted disease; intracellular obligate which closely resembles a gram negative bacteria; produces serious reproductive tract complications in either sex

Causes/Incidence

1.   *Chlamydia trachomatis*
2.   Most common bacterial STD in the United States
3.   Over 4 million infections annually
4.   Remains the most common cause of cervicitis and urethritis in adolescents

Signs/Symptoms

1.   Females: Often asymptomatic
      a.   Dysuria
      b.   Intramenstrual spotting
      c.   Postcoital bleeding
      d.   Dyspareunia
      e.   Vaginal discharge
      f.   Lower abdominal/pelvic pain
2.   Males: Often asymptomatic
      a.   Thick, cloudy, penile discharge
      b.   Dysuria
      c.   Testicular pain

Laboratory/Diagnostics

1.   Culture is most definitive but takes 3 to 9 days
2.   Enzyme immunoassay (EIA) for screening: Results in 30 to 120 minutes; low cost

Management

1.   Azithromycin (Zithromax) 1 gram orally in a single dose, or:
2.   Doxycycline (Vibromycin) 100 mg orally twice a day × 7 days
3.   Alternatives

a. Erythromycin 500 mg twice a day × 7 days for pregnant patients
b. Ofloxacin 300 mg orally twice day × 7 days
4. Report to the health department

Gonorrhea

A bacterial STD caused by *Neisseria gonorrheae* (gram negative diplococci); the organism may be cultured from the genitourinary tract, oropharynx, conjunctiva, and/or anorectum

Causes/Incidence

1. Causes urethritis in men and cervicitis in women
2. Leading cause of infertility among females
3. Occurs in 1 to 2% of the general population
4. Male-to-female transmission: 80 to 90% after exposure
5. Female-to-male transmission: 20% after exposure

Signs/Symptoms

1. Females are often asymptomatic (80%)
   a. Dysuria
   b. Urinary frequency
   c. Mucopurulent vaginal discharge
   d. Labial pain/swelling
   e. Lower abdominal pain
   f. Fever
   g. Abnormal menses
   h. Dysmenorrhea
   i. Nausea/vomiting
2. Males are often asymptomatic
   a. Dysuria
   b. Frequency
   c. White/yellow-green penile discharge
   d. Testicular pain

Laboratory/Diagnostics

1. Gram stain of discharge shows gram-negative diplococci and white blood cells (WBCs)
2. Cervical culture for *N. gonorrhoeae* using Thayer-Martin or Transgrow media

Management

1. Ceftriaxone (Rocephin) 125 mg intramuscular single dose
2. Co-treat for chlamydia
3. All contact should be treated
4. Report to the health department

Syphilis

A sexually transmitted disease involving multiple organ systems and caused by Treponema pallidum, a spirochete; the causative organism may be transmitted across the placenta

Incidence/Prevalence

1. Third most commonly-reported infectious disease in the U.S.
2. 200,000 new cases annually
3. Approximately 40,000 cases in the U.S. annually
4. Congenital syphilis occurs in about 1:10,000 pregnancies.
5. Incubation is 10 to 90 days

Signs/Symptoms

Clinical Stages

1. Primary
   a. Chancre present at site of inoculation 2 to 6 weeks after exposure
   b. Chancre indurated and painless
   c. Regional lymphadenopathy
2. Secondary
   a. Occurs 6 to 8 weeks later
   b. Flu-like symptoms
   c. Generalized lymphadenopathy
   d. Generalized maculopapular rash, especially on the palms and soles
3. Latent syphilis
   a. Seropositive, but asymptomatic
   b. About 1/3 of untreated cases develop tertiary syphilis
4. Tertiary
   a. Leukoplakia
   b. Cardiac insufficiency: Aortitis, aneurysms, aortic regurgitation
   c. Infiltrative tumors of skin, bones, liver
   d. Central nervous system (CNS) involvement: Meningitis, hemiparesis, hemiplegia, others

Diagnosis

1. Primary: Typical lesion or newly positive syphilis screen
   a. Dark field microscopy shows treponemes in 95% of chancres
2. Secondary: Clinical presentation with strongly reactive syphilis screen
3. Latent/Tertiary: Serologic evidence of untreated syphilis

Serologic Tests

1. Non-treponemal antibody tests include: Venereal Disease Research Laboratory (VDRL) and/or the Rapid Plasma Reagin (RPR)

2. Treponemal tests
   a. Fluorescent Treponemal Antibody Absorption (FTA-ABS): Following the non-treponemal screen, confirms positive in 85 to 95% of primary cases and 100% of secondary cases
   b. Microhemaglutination Assay for Antibody to Treponema Pallidum (MHA-TP)

Management

1. Primary, secondary, early latent of less than 1 year duration:
   a. Benzanthine penicillin G: 2.4 million units intramuscularly (IM)
2. Late, latent of indeterminate length, tertiary
   a. Benzanthine penicillin G: 2.4 million units IM weekly × 3 weeks
3. For penicillin allergic patients:
   a. Doxycycline 100 mg orally twice a day × 2 weeks, or:
   b. Erythromycin 500 mg four times a day × 2 weeks; requires careful follow-up
4. Report all cases to the health department
5. Follow-up at 3 and 6 months

Bacterial Vaginosis

A vaginal infection in which several species of bacteria interact to alter the vaginal flora

Causes/Incidence

1. Increased pH and decreased lactobacilli
2. Most prevalent vaginal infection in women of reproductive age
3. Not considered an STD/STI; seen more often in sexually active women

Signs/Symptoms

1. Increased milky discharge
2. May have pruritus
3. Malodorous "fishy" discharge most evident after sexual intercourse
4. Cervic/uterus/adnexa within normal limits

Laboratory/Diagnostics

1. Wet mount
   a. Clue cells: Epithelial cells stippled with bacteria
   b. Decreased/absent lactobacilli
   c. Few or absent WBC
2. Positive amine "whiff" test (fishy odor when potassium hydroxide (KOH) added to slide)
3. pH > 4.5 from lateral fornices

Treatment

1.   Metronidazole 2 gm in one dose (84% cure) or:
2.   Metronidazole 500 mg twice a day × 7 days (95% cure) or:
3.   Clindamycin 300 mg twice a day × 7 days or:
4.   Intravaginal metronidazole or clindamycin

Herpes

Recurrent, viral sexually transmitted disease that is associated with painful lesions

Causes

1.   Herpes simplex virus (HSV) type 1: Found on the lips, face, and mucosa
2.   HSV type 2: Found on the genitalia
3.   Transmission by direct contact with active lesions or by virus containing fluid (e.g., saliva or cervical secretions)

Signs/Symptoms

1.   Initial: Fever, malaise, dysuria, painful/pruritic ulcers for 12 days
2.   Recurrent: Less painful/pruritic ulcers for 5 days

Laboratory/Diagnostics

1.   Papanicolaou or Tzanck stain
2.   Viral culture is most definitive

Management

1.   No curative treatment
2.   Symptomatic treatment with drying and antipruritic agents
3.   Treatment options
        a.   Acyclovir (Zovirax): Topical, oral, IV ; pregnancy B; documented safety to 2 years of age..
        b.   Famciclovir
        c.   Valacyclovir: Especially useful for asymptomatic viral shedding of HSV-2

Acquired Immune Deficiency Syndrome (AIDS)

A disorder characterized by immunodeficiency as the result of infections by the human immune-deficiency virus (HIV)

Epidemiology

1.   Modes of transmission typically maternal infant perinatal transmission
2.   Breastfeeding is primary postnatal vertical route
3.   Average age of onset of perinatal infection is 8 to 9 months

Signs/Symptoms

1. Low birth weight
2. Recurrent infections
3. Diminishing activity
4. Developmental delay
5. Falling ratio of head circumference to height/weight
6. Generalized lymphadenopathy
7. Hepatosplenomegaly
8. Others

Laboratory/Diagnostics

1. Screening:
   a. In infants, HIV polymerase chain reaction (PCR) testing is used
   b. In older children, the enzyme-linked immunosorbent assay (ELISA) screening is used (sensitivity > 99.9%)
2. Confirmatory Testing:
   a. The western blot test is confirmatory
3. Absolute CD4 lymphocyte count: Normal > 800 cells/uL
4. CD4 lymphocyte percentage
   a. May be more accurate than the absolute CD4 count
   b. Risk of progression to AIDS high when < 20%
5. Viral load
   a. PCR based quantitative measure of number of copies of HIV branched DNA or ribonucleic acid (RNA)
   b. Results correlate closely with progression of HIV
   c. Drops dramatically in response to certain antiretroviral combinations
   d. Ideally, should be < 5000 copies, or "zero," or "undetectable"
6. Other related testing for associated conditions
   a. CBC
   b. Syphilis serology
   c. Hepatitis serology
   d. Toxoplasmosis serology
   e. Cytomegalovirus (CMV) serology
   f. PPD (> 5mm considered reactive)
   g. Pap smear
   h. Others

Management

1. Therapy for opportunistic infections
   a. Treat or refer as infections occur
   b. Bactrim for pneumocystis pneumonia (Pneumocystis jirovecii) prevention

    c. Consider the need for tuberculosis prophylaxis as needed

    d. Monitor for CMV which occurs in some patients

  2. Antiretroviral treatment

    a. Combination treatment: With highly active antiretroviral therapy (HAART) is standard

    b. Start no later than when the patient has a CD4 of 350 uL

    c. Drug resistance may develop rapidly; teach to take medications exactly as prescribed: At the same time every day

  3. Referral to an HIV infectious disease specialist

Sample Questions

1. Management of glomerulonephritis in the child includes numerous
    diagnostic tests. The most important for the practitioner to consider is the:
    a. Culture and sensitivity blood smear
    b. Test for streptococcus
    c. Examination for sexual abuse
    d. X-ray for kidney calculus

2. A newborn is checked in the nursery and found to have 1 undescended
    testis and hypospadias. You will take the following action:
    a. No action is necessary at this time.
    b. The testicle will need to be surgically brought down if it does not
        drop within 1 year.
    c. Order a chromosomal and endocrinological evaluation.
    d. Order serum luteinizing hormone, follicle-stimulating hormone,
        and testosterone tests.

3. Genital herpes is a sexually transmitted disease (STD) caused by the
    herpes simplex virus types 1 (HSV-1) and 2 (HSV-2). Which of the following
    is true of this disease?
    a. Most genital herpes is caused by HSV-1.
    b. When blisters break, they leave tender ulcers (sores) that may
        take 2 to 4 months to heal.
    c. The number of outbreaks number of outbreaks tends to increase
        over a period of years.
    d. Another outbreak can appear weeks or months after the first, but
        it almost always is less severe and shorter than the first outbreak.

Answers

1. Correct Answer: B
The most common cause is post infectious streptococcus species (group a, beta-hemolytic).

2. Correct Answer: C
Cryptorchidism: For the typical patient with a unilateral palpable or non-palpable undescended testis, no further laboratory evaluation is necessary. For the patient with bilateral undescended testis, with one testis palpable, no further workup is necessary. The patient with bilateral non-palpable testes should have a chromosomal and endocrinological evaluation, as should the patient with one or two undescended testes and hypospadias. If the patient has bilateral non-palpable testes and is less than 3 months of age, serum luteinizing hormone, follicle-stimulating hormone, and testosterone will determine whether testes are present. After that age, human chorionic gonadotropin stimulation will result in a measurable serum testosterone, if testes are present. A failure to respond to human chorionic gonadotropin stimulation in combination with elevated luteinizing hormone/follicle-stimulating hormone levels is consistent with anorchia.

3. Correct Answer: D
Genital herpes is a sexually transmitted disease (STD) caused by the herpes simplex viruses type 1 (HSV-1) or type 2 (HSV-2). Most genital herpes is caused by HSV-2. Most individuals have no or only minimal signs or symptoms from HSV-1 or HSV-2 infection. When signs do occur, they typically appear as one or more blisters on or around the genitals or rectum. The blisters break, leaving tender ulcers (sores) that may take two to four weeks to heal the first time they occur. Typically, another outbreak can appear weeks or months after the first, but it almost always is less severe and shorter than the first outbreak. Although the infection can stay in the body indefinitely, the number of outbreaks tends to decrease over a period of years.

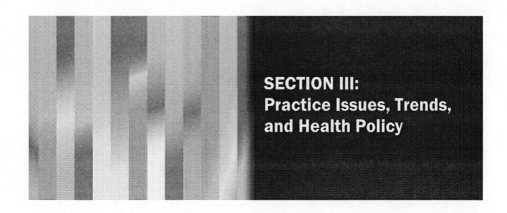

SECTION III:
Practice Issues, Trends,
and Health Policy

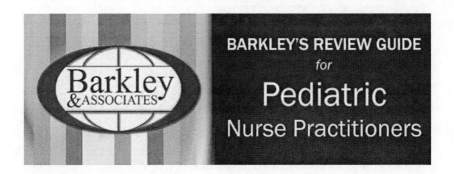

The Nurse Practitioner/Patient Relationship

Therapeutic Relationships

Establishing Rapport and Professional Therapeutic Relationships

1.   Non-judgmental approach
2.   Mutual trust
3.   Professional boundaries
4.   Confidentiality
5.   Cultural competency
     a.   Respect
     b.   Spiritual needs

Therapeutic Communication

1.   Listen more than talk
2.   "Tell me..."
3.   Never, "Why?"
4.   Focus on feelings
     a.   Mad, sad, glad, afraid, ashamed
5.   Do not mince words; no euphemisms
     a.   "I am concerned about alcoholism"
     b.   "I'm sorry, but she died"

Crisis Intervention

1.   Ensure safety and boundaries
     a.   Call the security office if necessary
2.   Establish trust and rapport

Crisis/Acute Grief Therapeutic Communication

1.   Acknowledge feelings
2.   Show empathy

Advanced Directives vs. Living Wills

1.   Advanced Directive: Written statement of a patient's intent regarding medical treatment
     a.   The Patient Self-Determination Act of 1990 requires that all patients entering a hospital should be advised of their right to execute an advanced directive

2. Healthcare Directive: Type of advanced directive that may (or may not) include a living will and/or specifications regarding durable power of attorney in one or two separate documents

3. Living Will: Written compilation of statements in document format that specifies which life-prolonging measures one does and does not want to be taken if he/she becomes incapacitated:

   a. In the United States, most states recognize living wills as long as the will is specific enough and addresses the problem at hand

   b. Living wills often include granting durable power of attorney to a significant other to act as a proxy/agent/attorney-in-fact for the patient in making healthcare decisions should the patient become incapacitated. Essentially, the proxy is responsible for articulating the patient's advanced directive

   c. Power of attorney must usually be in writing before it will be honored by most institutions such as hospitals, banks, etc.

Privacy and Confidentiality

Health Insurance Portability and Accountability Act (HIPAA)

1. Title I of HIPAA protects health insurance coverage for workers and their families when they change or lose their jobs

2. Title II of HIPAA, known as the Administrative Simplification (AS) provisions, requires the establishment of national standards for electronic health care transactions and national identifiers for providers, health insurance plans, and employers

   a. The Office for Civil Rights enforces the HIPAA, which protects the:
      i. Privacy of individually identifiable health information
      ii. HIPAA Security Rule, which sets national standards for the security of electronic protected health information
      iii. Confidentiality provisions of the Patient Safety Rule, which protect identifiable information being used to analyze patient safety events and improve patient safety

"Covered Entities" Required to Follow HIPAA Regulations

1. Health plans (health insurance companies, HMOs, company health plans, and certain government programs that pay for health care, such as Medicare and Medicaid)

2. Most health care providers (especially those who use electronic billing to health insurers)

3. Health care clearinghouses (those that process nonstandard health information data received from another entity into a standard, such as standard electronic formats)

Examples of HIPAA Protected Information

1. Written information in the medical record

2. Conversations among healthcare providers about one's care or treatment
3. Patient information stored in a health insurer's computer system
4. Patient billing information stored at a clinic
5. A patient's health information cannot be used or shared without written permission, unless this law allows it
6. Without a patient's written authorization, a provider generally cannot:
   a. Disclose information to one's employer
   b. Use or share a patient's information for marketing or advertising purposes
   c. Share private notes about a patient's health care

Entity Requirements to Protect Information

1. Safeguards must be in place to protect patients' health information
2. Reasonably limit use and provide minimum necessary disclosures to accomplish their intended purpose
3. Must ensure contracts are in place with contractors and others, ensuring that use and disclosure of health information is proper and safeguarded
4. Must have procedures in place to limit who can view and access health information, as well as implement training programs for employees about how to protect health information

The Privacy Rule: Patients' Rights

1. See or receive a copy of their health records
2. Have corrections added to their health information
3. Receive a notice that tells the patient how their health information may be used and shared
4. Decide if they want to give permission before their health information can be used or shared for certain purposes, such as for marketing
5. Receive a report outlining when and why their health information was shared for certain purposes
6. File complaints with one's healthcare provider, health insurer, and/or the U.S. government if their rights are being denied or if their health information is not being protected

Situations for Which Health Information Is Allowed to Be Viewed/Shared:

1. To ensure proper treatment and coordination of care
2. To pay for healthcare services (e.g., physicians, nurse practitioners (NPs), hospitals, etc.)
3. With a patient's family, relatives, friends, or others the patient identifies as being involved with their health care or bill payment (unless the patient objects)
4. To ensure quality care given by healthcare providers (e.g., physicians, NPs, nursing homes, etc.)
5. To protect the health of the public (e.g., reporting disease outbreaks)
6. To make required reports to the police (e.g., reporting gunshot wounds)

Examples of Those Not Required to Follow HIPAA

1. Life insurers
2. Employers
3. Workers compensation carriers
4. Many schools and school districts
5. Many state agencies like child protective service agencies
6. Many law enforcement agencies
7. Many municipal offices
8. Others

The Patient Safety and Quality Improvement Act (PSQIA)

1. Establishes a voluntary reporting system to enhance the data available to assess and resolve patient safety and health care quality issues
2. PSQIA provides federal privilege and confidentiality protections for patient safety information called patient safety work product to encourage the reporting and analysis of medical errors
   a. Patient safety work product includes information collected and created during the reporting and analysis of patient safety events
3. The confidentiality provisions should serve to improve patient safety outcomes by creating an environment where providers may report and examine patient safety events without fear of increased liability risk. The aim is that greater reporting and analysis of patient safety events will yield increased data and better understanding of patient safety events
4. The Agency for Healthcare Research and Quality (AHRQ) has additional responsibility for listing patient safety organizations (PSOs), which are external experts established by the Patient Safety Act to collect and analyze patient safety information

Confidentiality vs. "Duty to Warn"

1. The "Duty to Warn" supersedes the right to confidentiality if a patient's condition may endanger others
2. The duty to protect a patient from harming him/herself supersedes the right to confidentiality

Invasion of Privacy

1. Damaging one's reputation as a result of information being shared without the patient's permission
2. The charge cannot be made if the information can be shown to have been accurate, given in good faith, and the receiver had a valid reason for obtaining the information (e.g., a consulting practitioner has a right to know specific patient information)

Health Care Delivery

"Healthy People 2020"

1. Access to health care and improved health are both major issues for health policy
2. Continuance of Healthy People 2000; published in 1990 by the United States Department of Health and Human Services
3. Goals:
   a. Increase the quality and years of healthy life
   b. Eliminate health disparities among Americans
4. Document contains hundreds of health objectives based on numerous focus areas
5. Objectives relate to equal access, availability, cost, quality of care, etc.
6. Used to understand health status of the nation and plan prevention programs
7. Individuals, communities, and organizations are responsible for determining how to meet the goals of Healthy People 2020.

"Reporting" Statutes

Require practitioners to report specific health-related information; vary from state to state but commonly involve:

1. Criminal acts and injury from a dangerous weapon (police)
2. In most states, the NP must notify the Department of Health (DHHS) of the following diagnoses:
   a. Gonorrhea
   b. Chlamydia
   c. Syphilis
   d. HIV
   e. Tb
3. Animal bites (animal control; subsidiary of the DHHS)
4. Suspected or actual child or elder abuse (police via social services).
5. Domestic violence: NPs are not legally required to report in most states.

Collaborative Practice

1. Exists to enhance the quality of care and improve patient outcomes.
2. American Nurses Association (ANA's) Nursing: A Social Policy Statement (1995) describes collaboration as a "true partnership" in which all players have and desire power, share common goals, and recognize/accept separate areas of responsibility and activity."

Navigating the Health Care System for Patients

1. Social services
2. Psychiatric services
3. Police

277

4.   Security officers
5.   Physical therapy
6.   Occupational therapy

Issues Regarding Access to Care

1.   Home health
2.   Hospice
3.   Skilled nursing facilities
4.   Private duty nursing

Health Care Financing

1.   Coding: Evaluation and Management (E&M) codes identify the level of care provided
    a.   Codes match the level of service provided to the complexity of the presenting patient problem.
2.   Billing
3.   Reimbursement
4.   Third party payers

Categories of Third-Party Payers

1.   Medicare
2.   Medicaid
3.   Commercial indemnity insurers
4.   Commercial management organizations such as health maintenance organizations (HMOs).
5.   Businesses or schools wanting health services for employees or students.

Appropriate Level Physical Exam Documentation to Determine Levels of E/M Services

1.   Problem focused: a limited examination of the affected body area or organ system.
2.   Expanded problem focused: a limited examination of the affected body area or organ system and any other symptomatic or related body areas or organ systems.
3.   Detailed: an extended examination of the affected body areas or organ systems and any other symptomatic or related body areas or organ systems.
4.   Comprehensive: a general multi-system examination, or complete examination of a single organ system and other symptomatic or related body areas or organ systems.

Types of Medicare

1.   Medicare A: covers inpatient/hospitalization, skilled nursing facility services, home health services and/or hospice associated with the

inpatient event; most individuals qualify to receive benefits at 65 years of age.
2.   Medicare B: covers physician services, outpatient hospital services, laboratory and diagnostic procedures, medical equipment, and some home health services.
    a.   Supplemental medical insurance requires recipients to pay a premium
    b.   NPs and clinical nurse specialists (CNSs) receive 85% of physician reimbursement for services provided in collaboration with a physician.
3.   Medicare C: "A + B = C"
    a.   Formerly known as "Medicare+Choice" is now known as "Medicare Advantage."
    b.   Patients entitled to Medicare Part A and enrolled in Part B, are eligible to receive all of their health care services through one of the provider organizations under Part C (such as HMOs, PPOs, etc.).
4.   Medicare D: limited prescription drug coverage
    a.   Plans offered by insurance and other private companies are approved by Medicare.
    b.   Monthly premium required.
    c.   Co-pay on each prescription is required.
    d.   Penalty may be applicable if not enrolled when first eligible; assistance is available for people with limited income and resources.

Examples of NP Billing under Medicare B, described by a Current Procedural Terminology (CPT) code and an International Classification of Disease, 9th Edition (ICD-9) code:

1.   Diagnosis
2.   Therapy
3.   Surgery consultation
4.   Care plan oversight

Services That Do Not Meet Medicare's Definition of Physician Services:

1.   Regular physical exams
2.   Health maintenance screenings
3.   Counseling for well patients
4.   Others (http://www.medicare.gov/Contacts/Home.asp)

Medicare Rules for Nurse Practitioners

1.   To qualify to be a Medicare provider, an NP must:
    a.   Hold a state license as an NP
    b.   Be certified as an NP by a recognized national certifying body

     c.   Hold at least an MSN degree
2.   The NP meets Medicare qualification requirements
     a.   The practice/facility accepts Medicare payment (i.e., 85% of physician schedule rate for bills submitted under the NP's provider number)
3.   No facility or other provider charges or is paid with respect to the furnishing of services.
4.   The services are:
     a.   "Physician services": those for which a physician can bill Medicare.
     b.   Performed in collaboration with a physician
     c.   Within the NP's scope of practice as defined by state law.

Medicare Payments

1.   Medicare pays 80% of the patient's bill for physician services, and the patient pays 20%.
2.   Medicare reimburses NPs 85% of the physician fee delineated in Medicare's Physician Fee Schedule.
3.   For a procedure, Medicare pays NPs 80% of the 85% of the Physician Fee Schedule rate.
4.   Practices must bill under the provider of the clinician who performs a given service. The exception is "incident-to" billing. When billing "incident to" a physician's service, a practice may be reimbursed 100% of the Physician Fee Schedule rate.

Incident-to Billing

Services billed under the physician's provider number to get the full physician fee (100%) given the following rules:

1.   The services are:
     a.   An integral, although incidental, part of the physician's professional service
     b.   Commonly rendered without charge or included in the physician's bill.
     c.   Of a type commonly furnished in physician's offices or clinics.
     d.   Furnished under the physician's direct personal supervision and are furnished by the physician or by an individual who is an employee or independent contractor of the physician. Direct supervision does not require the physician's presence in the same room but the physician must be present in the same office suite and immediately available.
     e.   The physician must perform "the initial service and subsequent services of a frequency which reflect his or her active participation in the management of the course of treatment."

2. The physician or other provider under whose name and number the bill is submitted must be the individual present in the office suite when the service is provided.
3. Incident-to billing is not allowed in the hospital setting; an NP must bill under his/her provider number.
4. A nurse practitioner may bill for an assistant's work (performing an EKG for example) under the NP's provider number as long as the rules for incident-to billing are followed.

Other Rules for Billing

1. Physicians and NPs may see a patient on the same day for their services; however, the two must coordinate billing to avoid duplicate payments.
2. For inpatients, physicians and NPs must decide for which party (the NP or the physician) should bill, given the amount of services rendered by each on given day.
3. For home NP visits billable for Medicare A services, NPs do not need a physician's order to bill under the NP's provider number, unless the NP is providing nursing services exclusively

Medicaid

A federally supported, state administered program for low-income families and individuals:

1. Benefits vary from state to state.
2. Medicaid payments are made after other insurance or third party payments have been made.

Case Management

1. Involves a comprehensive and systematic approach to provide quality care.
2. Purpose: mobilize, monitor and control resources that a patient uses during a course of an illness while balancing quality and cost.

Quality Assurance (QA)/Quality Improvement (QI)/Continuous Process Improvement (CPI)

1. A management process of monitoring, evaluating, continuous review, and improving the quality in providing health care.
2. Quality assurance: a process for evaluating the care of patients using established standards of care to ensure quality.
3. Based on the methodology developed by Deming and tested in Japanese industry that quality can be improved by continually monitoring structure, process and outcome standards (CQI).
   a. Structures: inputs into care such as resources, equipment, or numbers and qualifications of staff.

      b.   Processes of care: includes assessments, planning, performing treatments and managing complications.

      c.   Outcomes: include complications, adverse events, short term results of treatment and long term results of patient health and functioning.

4.   Used to assess, monitor, and improve care provided to patients.

5.   Components include monitoring of care quality, care appropriateness, effectiveness of care, cost of care, self-regulation and peer review to ensure compliance to care standards.

6.   Steps of Continuous Quality Improvement/Quality Assurance (outlined by the Joint Commission)

      a.   Quality planning (i.e., developing a quality management plan which assigns responsibility for degree of involvement).

      b.   Delineates scope of care.

7.   Identify important aspects of care.

8.   Identify indicators related to aspects of care.

      a.   Establish thresholds for evaluation related to the indicators.

      b.   Collect and organize data

      c.   Evaluate care when thresholds are reached

      d.   Take action to improve care

      e.   Assess the effectiveness of the action and document improvement.

      f.   Communicate relevant information.

9.   Critical Path: Contains key patient care activities and time frames for those activities which are needed for a specific case type or diagnosis-related group (DRG)

10.   Care Map: A newer version of the critical path and is a blueprint for planning and managing care delivered by all disciplines:

      a.   The Care Map contains a critical path section plus a section that identifies common problems encountered by patients of a specific case type, the day-to-day goals that the patient must achieve, and the final desired clinical outcomes.

      b.   Monitoring of outcomes of care is a very important goal.

Sentinel Events

1.   Unexpected occurrences involving death or serious physical or psychological injury, or the risk thereof

2.   Serious injury specifically includes loss of limb or function.

3.   The phrase, "or the risk thereof" includes any process variation for which a recurrence would carry a significant chance of a serious adverse outcome.

4.   Such events are called "sentinel" because these signal the need for immediate investigation and response.

5.   The terms "sentinel event" and "medical error" are not synonymous; not all sentinel events occur because of an error and not all errors result in sentinel events.
6.   In response to a sentinel event (e.g., falls in nursing homes or a colleague's behavior that undermines a culture of safety), clinicians and institutions are expected to conduct a root cause analysis.

Root Cause Analysis

A tool for identifying prevention strategies to ensure safety

1.   A process that is part of the effort to build a culture of safety and move beyond the culture of blame
2.   Involves and incorporates:
   a.   Inter-disciplinary experts from the frontline services.
   b.   Those who are the most familiar with a situation.
   c.   Continually digging deeper by asking why, why, why at each level of cause and effect.
   d.   Identifying changes that need to be made to systems.
   e.   A process that is as impartial as possible.

Professional Responsibility

Scope of Practice
1.   Based on legal allowances in each State, according to and delineated by individual State Nurse Practice Acts
2.   Provides guidelines for nursing practice; varies from state to state.
3.   Key elements of the NP role include integration of care across the acute illness continuum with collaboration and coordination of care, research-based clinical practice, clinical leadership, family assessment and discharge planning.

Standards of Advanced Practice
1.   Delineated by the American Nurses Association (1996) as authoritative statements by which to measure quality of practice, service, or education.
2.   Both generic and specific specialty standards exist.

State Practice Acts
1.   Authorize Boards of Nursing in each state to establish statutory authority for licensure of registered nurses.
2.   Authority includes use of title, authorization for scope of practice including prescriptive authority, and disciplinary grounds.
3.   States also vary in specific practice requirements, such as certification.

Prescriptive Authority

1.   The ability and extent of the NP's ability to prescribe medications to patients is dependent on state nurse practice acts.
2.   While the Drug Enforcement Agency (DEA) has ruled that nurses in advanced practice may obtain registration numbers, state practice acts dictate the level of prescriptive authority allowed.

Credentials

1.   Encompass required education, licensure and certification to practice as a nurse practitioner.
2.   Establish minimal levels of acceptable performance.
3.   Credentialing is necessary to:
      a.   Ensure that safe health care is provided by qualified individuals
      b.   Comply with federal and state laws relating to advanced practice nursing
4.   Acknowledges the scope of practice of the NP
5.   Mandates accountability
6.   Enforces professional standards for practice

Licensure

1.   Establishes that a person is qualified to perform in a particular professional role.
2.   Licensure is granted as defined by rules and regulations set forth by a governmental regulatory body (i.e., state board of nursing).

Certification

1.   Establishes that a person has met certain standards in a particular profession which signify mastery of specialized knowledge and skills.
2.   Certification is granted by nongovernmental agencies such as the American Nurses Credentialing Center (ANCC), American Academy of Nurse Practitioners (AANP) , Pediatric Nursing Certification Board (PNCB), National Certification Corporation (NCC).

Admitting Privileges to Hospitals

1.   Non-physician providers were granted the possibility of hospital staff membership in 1983 by the Joint Commission.

Credentialing and Privileging

1.   Process by which a nurse practitioner is granted permission to practice in an inpatient setting.
2.   Credentialing with hospital privileges is granted by a Hospital Credentialing Committee comprised of physicians who hold privileges at the given hospital where the NP has made request.
3.   Privileges may be granted in part or full; stipulations regarding the allowance of future privileges may be made by the Credentialing

Committee (a number of additional supervised hours required before a certain privilege is granted).

Patient Medical Abandonment

1. Results when the caregiver-patient relationship is terminated without making reasonable arrangements with an appropriate person so that care by others can be continued.
2. Determination of patient abandonment may depend on many factors including:
    a. Whether the practitioner accepted the patient assignment (which formally created a practitioner-patient relationship).
    b. Whether the practitioner provided reasonable notice before terminating the practitioner-patient relationship.
    c. Whether reasonable arrangements could have been made to continue patient care when the adequate notification was given.

3. In most cases, the following does not constitute patient abandonment:
    a. An NP refuses to accept responsibility for a patient assignment when the NP has given reasonable notice to the proper authority that the NP lacks competence to carry out the assignment.
    b. An NP refuses an assignment of a double shift or additional hours beyond the posted work schedule when proper notification has been given.
4. When "proper notification has been given" potentially becomes a problematic and sometimes, arguable phrase in difference of opinion.

Risk Management

1. A systematic effort to reduce risk begins with a formal, written risk management plan that includes:
    a. The organization's goals.
    b. Delineation of the program's scope, components and methods.
    c. Delegating responsibility for implementation and enforcement.
    d. Demonstrating commitment by the board
    e. Articulates guarantees of confidentiality and immunity from retaliation for those who report sensitive information.
2. Incident reports: the most common method of documentation.
3. Policies regarding incident reports should address:
    a. Persons authorized to complete a report
    b. Persons responsible for review a report
    c. Immediate actions needed to minimize the effects of the report's event.
    d. Persons responsible for follow-up.
    e. A plan for monitoring the aftermath of the report's event.

      f.   Security and storage of completed incident report forms.

4.   Satisfaction surveys: important form for identifying problems before developing into actual incidents or claims; important to track and analyze just like incident reports:

      a.   Patient satisfaction surveys.

      b.   Employee and/or practitioner satisfaction surveys.

5.   Complaints: a key source of potential risk management information. A risk management plan should delineate tracking, analyzing and managing complaints by clearly identifying:

      a.   Persons notified after receiving a complaint

      b.   Persons responsible for responding to the complaint.

      c.   Persons responsible for monitoring follow-up resolution of the complaint.

6.   Action taking initiatives:

      a.   Prevention: proactive risk awareness and safety programs in place..

      b.   Correction: post-incident remediation to minimize the impact and prevent future occurrences.

7.   Corrective steps must be monitored and audited

      a.   Documentation: essential for legal defense; thorough medical records and institutional policies.

      b.   Education: In-services of all staff at orientation and annually, at a minimum.

      c.   Departmental coordination: encouraging departments and managers to work together for the common goal of improved patient and staff safety.

Medical Futility

1.   Refers to interventions that are unlikely to produce any significant benefit for the patient; "Does the intervention have any reasonable prospect of helping this patient?

2.   Two kinds of medical futility are often distinguished:

      a.   Quantitative futility: where the likelihood that an intervention will benefit the patient is extremely poor, and

      b.   Qualitative futility: where the quality of benefit an intervention will produce is extremely poor.

Informed Consent and Obtaining Informed Consent

1.   Competence (Decisional Capability): a state in which a patient is able to make personal decisions about his or her care:

      a.   Implies the ability to understand, reason, differentiate good and bad and communicate.

2.   Informed Consent: a state indicating that a patient has received adequate instruction or information regarding aspects of care to make a prudent, personal choice regarding such treatment.
    a.   Includes discussing all of the benefits and risks with a patient in order to make a truly informed decision.
    b.   Generally, consent is assumed if the patient's condition is life-threatening.
3.   Right to Refuse Care: Patients must be advised at the time of their admission to a federally funded institution such as a hospital, nursing home, hospice, HMO, etc. that they have a right to refuse care (Danforth Amendment, 1991).
    a.   Care that may be refused includes any, some, or all, as long as the patient has decisional capability (competence).

Ethical Principles

Ethics is the study of moral conduct and behavior which serves to govern conduct, thereby protecting the rights of an individual

Key Ethical Principles

1.   Nonmaleficence: The duty to do no harm
2.   Utilitarianism: The right act is the one that produces the greatest good for the greatest number
3.   Beneficence: The duty to prevent harm and promote good
4.   Justice: The duty to be fair
5.   Fidelity: The duty to be faithful
6.   Veracity: The duty to be truthful
7.   Autonomy: The duty to respect an individual's thoughts and actions

Dismissing/Discharging a Patient or Closing a Practice

1.   An NP cannot withdraw from caring for a patient without notification.
2.   Examples of reasons for discharging a patient from practice include: abuse from the patient, refusal to pay for services, or patients' persistent non-adherence to recommended care.
3.   Steps for discharging a patient from a practice:
    a.   Send a certified letter with return receipt requested; copy for the chart.
    b.   The content of letter should be general versus specific.
4.   The NP's practice should have established policies that all patients consent to in writing such as recommended care, including timeframes for canceling appointments or rescheduling and payment of services.
5.   These may serve as the foundation for the termination of healthcare:
    a.   Provide general healthcare coverage for the first 15 to 30 days post-termination deadline

   b.   Obtain release of information to provide copies of all needed records for the subsequent care provider.
6.   Obligations in closing a practice due to relocation, retirement or other changes:
   a.   Give the patient adequate time to find another provider
   b.   Keep all files for a minimum of five years. Follow state laws regarding storage requirements.
   c.   To avoid complaints of patient abandonment, provide timely notification and names of other providers and resources for future care

History of the Nurse Practitioner Role

1.   The role of the NP developed in the early 1960s as a result of physician shortages in the area of pediatrics.
2.   The first NP program was a pediatric NP program, begun in 1964, by Dr. Loretta Ford and Dr. Henry Silver at the University of Colorado Health Sciences Center
3.   Growth of NP programs soon ensued with distribution of NPs in various practice settings with an emphasis on ambulatory and outpatient care.
4.   The historical service of NPs in primary care resulted in part from the availability of federal funding for preventative and primary care NP education.
5.   Movement of NPs expanded to the inpatient setting as a result of managed care, hospital restructuring and decreases in medical residency programs.
6.   Four distinct roles for the nurse practitioner include expert:
   a.   Clinician
   b.   Consultant/collaborator
   c.   Educator
   d.   Researcher

Evidence-based Practice and Research Methods:

Major Steps in the Research Process

1.   Formulating the research problem
2.   Reviewing related literature
3.   Formulating the hypotheses
4.   Selecting the research design
5.   Identifying the population to be studied
6.   Specifying methods of data collection
7.   Designing the study
8.   Conducting the study
9.   Analyzing the data
10.   Interpreting the results

11.   Communicating the findings

Types of Research

1.   Non-experimental: a "no experiment" design; usually includes two broad categories of research, descriptive and ex post facto/correlational research:

    a.   Descriptive research: aims to describe situations, experiences, and phenomena as they exist.

    b.   Ex post facto or correlational research: examines relationships among variables

    c.   Other possibilities.

2.   Cross sectional: study that examines a population with a very similar attribute but differs in one specific variable (such as age) is designed to find relationships between variables at a specific point in time or "surveys."

3.   Cohort: Research study that compares a particular outcome (such as lung cancer) in groups of individuals who are alike in many ways but differ by a certain characteristic (e.g., female nurses who smoke compared with those who do not smoke).

4.   Longitudinal: A study that involves taking multiple measures of a group/population over an extended period of time to find relationships between variables.

5.   Experimental: Includes experimental manipulation of variables utilizing randomization and a control group to test the effects of an intervention or experiment:

    a.   Quasi-experimental research involves manipulation of variables but lacks a comparison group or randomization.

6.   Qualitative: includes case studies, open-ended questions, field studies, participant observation and ethnographic studies, where observations and interview techniques are used to explore phenomena through detailed descriptions of people, events, situations, or observed behavior:

    a.   Researcher bias is a potential problem.

    b.   Calls into question the generalizability of the findings.

    c.   Produces very rich data through no other means of research.

Research Terms

1.   Confidence interval: an interval, with limits at either end, with a specified probability of including the parameter being estimated:

    a.   A small confidence interval implies a very precise range of values.

    b.   Example: Confidence interval = 2.8-3.2 □ terminally ill bone cancer patients in the final stage of illness have between 2.8 and 3.2 episodes of nausea every 24 hours.

2.   Standard deviation (SD): indicates the average amount of deviation of values from the mean.

3. 66.6% of the sample falls within one SD of the mean
4. 95% of the sample falls within two SDs of the mean
    a. Level of significance: The probability level of which the results of statistical analyses are judged to indicate a statistically significant differences between groups:
        i. The probability of false rejection of the null hypothesis in a statistical test.
        ii. Example: probability is less than .05 of the experimental and control groups are considered to be significantly different.
    b. Perfect correlation: A measure of the interdependence of two random variables that ranges in value from -1 to +1
        i. -1 indicates a perfect negative correlation.
        ii. 0 indicates an absence of correlation.
    c. +1 indicates a perfect positive correlation.
5. T-test: Statistical test to evaluate the differences in means between two groups.
6. Reliability: The consistency of a measurement, or the degree to which an instrument measures the same way over time with the same subjects.
    a. Reflects the estimated repeatability of a measurement.
    b. A measure is considered reliable if a person's score on the same test given twice is similar.
    c. Reliability is estimated in two ways:
7. Test/retest: The more conservative method to estimate reliability:
    a. One should get the same score on exam 1 as one does on exam 2.
8. Internal consistency: Estimates reliability by grouping questions in a questionnaire that measure the same concept:
    a. Example: One could write two sets of three questions that measure the same concept (say knowledge of lipid panels) and after collecting the responses, runs a correlation between those two groups of 3 questions to determine if the instrument is reliably measuring that concept.
    b. Cronbach's alpha is a common way of computing correlation values among the questions on instruments. As with a correlation coefficient, the closer it is to one (optimal is more than .70), the higher the reliability estimate of the instrument.
    c. The major difference between test/retest and internal consistency estimates of reliability is that test/retest involves two administrations of the measurement instrument, whereas the internal consistency method involves only one.
9. Validity: The degree to which a variable measures what it is intended to measure.

Legal Terms

Liability

1. The legal responsibility that a nurse practitioner has for actions that fail to meet the standard of care, resulting in actual or potential harm to a patient.
2. Standards of care are used as criteria to measure whether negligence has occurred.

Negligence

1. Failure of an individual to do what a reasonable person would do, resulting in injury to the patient.

Malpractice

1. Failure of a professional to render services with the degree of care, diligence, and precaution that another member of the same profession under similar circumstances would render to prevent injury to someone else.
2. Malpractice may involve:
   a. Professional misconduct
   b. Unreasonable lack of skill
   c. Illegal/immoral conduct
   d. Other allegations resulting in harm to a patient
3. Malpractice insurance does not cover an advanced practice nurse (APN) from charges of practicing medicine without a license if the APN is practicing outside the legal scope of practice for that state.

Assault

1. An intentional act by one person that creates an apprehension in another of an imminent harmful or offensive contact:
   a. An assault is carried out by a threat of bodily harm coupled with an apparent, present ability to cause the harm.
   b. Examples: Shaking a fist in the air in the direction of another person, making the motion to inject someone against his will, etc.

Battery

1. An illegal, willful, angry, violent, or negligent striking of a person, his clothes, or anything with which he is in contact.
2. One can commit battery on an unconscious person, but not assault.

Defamation

1. A communication that causes someone to suffer a damaged reputation:
   a. Libel: Defaming, distributed written material
   b. Slander: Spoken defamation (spoken to other than the defamed party).

Involuntary Commitment

1.   In most states, there is a duty to commit someone who is in danger of hurting himself or others as a result of mental illness (e.g., patients who attempt suicide).
2.   A nurse practitioner is potentially liable if a patient is discharged while in danger of hurting himself or others.

Use of Restraints

1.   It is legal to forcefully restrain someone to prevent a patient from harming himself or others.
2.   The NP must document the exact reason/rational for why restraints are being ordered.
3.   An NP may be liable if excessive restraints are employed, the exact reason for using restraints is not documented, or safety checks of the restraints are not charted.

Good Samaritan Statutes

1.   Protect health care providers from law suits who aid at the scene of an accident and render reasonable, emergency care, within the NP's scope of practice.

Cultural Competence

Standards of Practice for Culturally Competent Nursing Care

Standard 1: Social Justice

Principles of social justice guide nurses' decisions related to the patient, family, community and other healthcare professionals. Nurses will develop leadership skills to advocate for socially just policies.

Standard 2: Critical Reflection

Engage in critical reflection of one's own values, beliefs and cultural heritage in order to have an awareness of how these qualities and issues can impact culturally congruent nursing care.

Standard 3: Transcultural Nursing Knowledge

Understand the perspectives, traditions, values, practices and family systems of culturally diverse individuals, families, communities and populations care for, as well as knowledge of complexities of achieving health and well-being.

Standard 4: Cross Cultural Practice

Utilize cross cultural knowledge and culturally sensitive skills implementing culturally congruent care.

Standard 5: Healthcare Systems and Organizations

Provide the resources and structure to evaluate and meet cultural and language needs of diverse clients.

Standard 6: Patient Advocacy and Empowerment

Recognize the effect of healthcare policies, delivery systems and resources on patient population and advocate and empower their patients.

Standard 7: Multicultural Workforce

Be activists for a more multicultural workforce in healthcare settings globally.

Standard 8: Education and Training

Be educationally prepared and receive ongoing continuing education in the knowledge and skills for nursing care that is culturally congruent, that is also included in the global health care agenda.

Standard 9: Cross Cultural Communication

Use effective, competent, communication with clients that consider verbal and non-verbal language, cultural values and context, and unique healthcare needs and perceptions.

Standard 10: Cross Cultural Leadership

Be able to influence individuals, groups and systems to achieve culturally competent outcomes for diverse populations.

Standard 11: Policy Development

Work with public/private organizations, professional associations and communities to establish policies and standards for comprehensive implementation and evaluation of culturally competent care.

Standard 12: Evidenced-Based Practice and Research

Practice is based on effective interventions for culturally diverse populations. Where lack of evidence exists, nurse researchers should test and investigate to contribute to reducing racial and ethnic inequalities in health outcomes.

Culturally and Linguistically Appropriate Services (CLAS)

1.   Ultimately, the aim of the standards is to contribute to the elimination of racial and ethnic health disparities and to improve the health of all Americans.
2.   There are 14 CLAS standards. The following standards guide all providers, including NPs, in their direct care roles.
   a.   Standard 4: Healthcare organizations must offer and provide language assistance services, including bilingual staff and

interpreter services, at no cost to each patient/consumer with limited English proficiency at all points of contact, in a timely manner during all hours of operation.

b.   Standard 5: Healthcare organizations must provide to patients/consumers in their preferred language, both verbal offers and written notices informing them of their rights to receive language assistance services.

c.   Standard 6: Healthcare organizations must assure the competence of language assistance provided to limited English proficient patients/consumers by interpreters and bilingual staff. Family and friends should not be used to provide interpretation services (except upon request by the patient/consumer)

Sample Questions

1. Root cause analysis is a process that is part of the effort to build a culture of safety and includes:

    a. Digging deeper into "Why?" at each level of cause and effect to eliminate fraud and dishonest providers by determination of human error
    b. Participation by the leadership of the organization and those most closely involved in the processes and systems
    c. A process that is as impartial as possible even though it may be obvious who or what is to blame
    d. Creating a "big picture" of the major problems within the system

2. In statistical significance testing, the p-value is the probability of obtaining a test statistic at least as extreme as the one that was actually observed; assuming that the null hypothesis is true. When the p-value is low, it means:

    a. The lower p-value, the more likely the result is if the null hypothesis is true.
    b. If the p-value is less than 0.05 or 0.01, one accepts the null hypothesis.
    c. If the p-value is less than 0.05 or 0.0, then the null is true.
    d. The lower p-value, the less likely the result is if the null hypothesis is true.

3. State Practice Acts regulate nurse practitioners by administering the following elements:

    a. The Nurse Practice Act legislated in each state of the U.S. specifically delineates requirements for registered nurses in advanced practice roles.
    b. The degree of legal authority for advanced practice nurses (APNs) to practice varies by state
    c. Prescriptive authority and reimbursement are controlled by the state.
    d. All are true.

Answers

1. Correct Answer: B

Root Cause Analysis is a tool for identifying prevention strategies to ensure safety.

1. A process that is part of the effort to build a culture of safety and move beyond the culture of blame
2. Involves and incorporates:
   a. Inter-disciplinary experts from the frontline services
   b. Those who are the most familiar with a situation
   c. Continually digging deeper by asking why, why, why at each level of cause and effect
   d. Identifying changes that need to be made to systems
   e. A process that is as impartial as possible
3. To be thorough, a root cause analysis must include:
   a. Determination of human and other factors
   b. Determination of related processes and systems
   c. Analysis of underlying cause and defect systems through a series of why questioning
   d. Identification of risks and their potential contributions
   e. Determination of potential improvement in processes or systems
4. To be credible, a root cause analysis must:
   a. Include participation by the leadership of the organization and those most closely
   b. Involved in the processes and systems
   c. Be internally consistent
   d. Include consideration of relevant literature
   e. Use the facts and ask "so what?" to determine all the possible consequences of a fact
   f. Include 5 Whys: Ask, "Why?" until you get to the root of the problem
   g. Drill down: Break down a problem into small, detailed parts to better understand the big picture
   h. Create cause-and-effect diagrams: Chart all possible causal factors to see where the trouble may have begun

2. Correct Answer: D

In statistical significance testing, the p-value is the probability of obtaining a test statistic at least as extreme as the one that was actually observed, assuming that the null hypothesis is true. The lower the p-value, the less likely the result is if the null hypothesis is true, and consequently the more "significant" the result is, in the sense of statistical significance. One often accepts the alternative hypothesis, (rejects a null hypothesis) if the p-value is less than 0.05 or 0.01, corresponding respectively to a 5% or 1% chance of rejecting the null hypothesis when it is true (Type I error).

3. Correct Answer: B

The degree of legal authority for Advanced Nurse Practitioners (APN) to practice varies by state. The Nurse Practice Act legislated in each state of the U.S. specifically delineates requirements for registered nurses in advanced practice roles. While registered nurses are now legally authorized to provide services for primary health promotion, disease prevention, and assessment of health status, questions remain as to the degree of independence, prescriptive authority, and reimbursement for APN for services. A broader definition of the scope of NP practice would enable expansion of primary care services to better serve the health care needs of the nation.

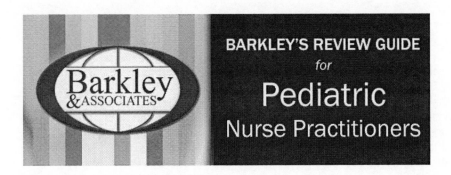

Index

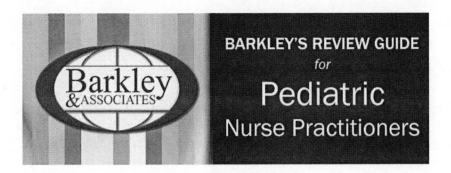

Bibliography

Acello, B. (2009). *The long-term care nursing desk reference.* Marblehead, MA: HCPro, Inc. /Opus Communications.

Aktan, N. M. (2010). *Fast facts for the new nurse practitioner: What you really need to know in a nutshell.* New York, NY: Springer Publishing Company.

Allen, P. J., Vessey, J. A. (2010). *Primary care of the child with a chronic condition* (5th ed.). St. Louis, MO: Mosby.

Allender, J. A. (2010). *Community health nursing promoting and protecting the public's health* (7th ed.). Philadelphia, PA: Lippincott Williams & Wilkins.

American Academy of Pediatrics. (2009). *Red book: Report of the committee on infectious diseases.* Washington, DC: Author.

American Academy of Pediatrics and the American Academy of Family Physicians Subcommittee on Management of Acute Otitis Media. (2004). Clinical practice guideline: Diagnosis and management of acute otitis media. *Pediatrics, 113*(5), 1451-1565.

American Academy of Pediatrics. (2011). *Recommended childhood and adolescent immunization schedule– United States, year 2011.* Retrieved from http://www.AAP.org/immunization.

American Academy of Pediatrics Red Book. (2009). *Report of the committee on infectious diseases* (28th ed.). Elk Grove, IL: American Academy of Pediatrics.

American Academy of Pediatrics. (2009). *Caring for your baby and young child: Birth to age 5* (5th ed.). New York, NY: Bantam Books.

American Academy of Pediatrics Subcommittee on Hyperbilirubinemia. (2004). Clinical practice guideline: Management of hyperbilirubinemia in the newborn infant 35 or more weeks of gestation. *Pediatrics, 114,* 207-316.

American Diabetes Association. (2007). Standards of medical care in diabetics – 2007. *Diabetes Care, 40,* S4-S41.

American Diabetes Association. (2009). Clinical practice recommendations – 2009. *Diabetes Care, 32*(1), S1-S97.

American Nurses Association. (2010). *Code of ethics for nurses with interpretive statements.* Washington, DC: American Nurses Publishing.

American Nurses Association. (2004). *Scope and standards of advanced practice registered nursing.* Washington, DC: American Nurses Publishing.

Anderson, B. J., Craig, A. S., Farley, M. M., Griffin, M. R., Hadler, J. L., Harrison, L. H., et al. (2006). Invasive pneumococcal disease among infants before and after introduction of pneumococcal conjugate vaccine. *Journal of the American Medical Association, 295*(14), 1668-1674.

Baid, H. (2006). Differential diagnosis in advanced nursing practice. *British Journal of Nursing, 15*(18), 1007-1011.

Balding, W. A., Burke, H., Corbett, S., Hall, J., Lyle, D. M., Phillips, A. R., & Stokes, D. (2006). Dealing with lead in Broken Hill– trends in blood leads levels in young children 1991-2003. *Science of the Total Environment, 359*(1-3), 111-119.

Barker, L. R., Fieback N. H., Kern D. E., Thomas, P. A., & Ziegelstein, R. C. (2006). *Principles of ambulatory medicine* (7th ed.). Baltimore, MD: Lippincott Williams & Wilkins.

Barkley, Jr. T. (2008). Cardiovascular assessment. In T. W. Barkley, Jr. & C. M. Myers (Eds.), *Practice guidelines for acute care nurse practitioners* (2nd ed., pp. 91-94). St. Louis, MO: Elsevier.

Barkley, Jr., T. (2008). Diabetes mellitus. In T. W. Barkley, Jr. & C. M. Myers (Eds.), *Practice guidelines for acute care nurse practitioners* (2nd ed., pp.447-462). St. Louis, MO: Elsevier.

Barkley, Jr., T. (2008). Differential diagnosis of pulmonary disorders. In T. W. Barkley, Jr. & C. M. Myers (Eds.), *Practice guidelines for acute care nurse practitioners* (2nd ed., pp. 253-258). St. Louis, MO: Elsevier.

Barkley, Jr. T. (2008). Inflammatory cardiac diseases. In T. W. Barkley, Jr. & C. M. Myers (Eds.), *Practice guidelines for acute care nurse practitioners* (2nd ed., pp. 163-168). St. Louis, MO: Elsevier.

Barkley, Jr., T. (2008). Lower respiratory tract pathogens. In T. W. Barkley, Jr. & C. M. Myers (Eds.), *Practice guidelines for acute care nurse practitioners* (2nd ed., pp. 313-322). St. Louis, MO: Elsevier.

Barkley, Jr., T. (2008). Pathophysiologically derived therapy for respiratory dysfunction. In T. W. Barkley, Jr. & C. M. Myers (Eds.), *Practice guidelines for acute care nurse practitioners* (2nd ed., pp. 292-295). St. Louis, MO: Elsevier.

Barkley, Jr. T. (2008). Thyroid disease. In T. W. Barkley, Jr. & C. M. Myers (Eds.), *Practice guidelines for acute care nurse practitioners* (2nd ed., pp.469-475). St. Louis, MO: Elsevier.

Barkley, Jr., T., Fortenberry, D. R., & Field, G. (2008). Obstructive (ventilatory) lung diseases. In T. W. Barkley, Jr. & C. M. Myers (Eds.), *Practice guidelines for acute care nurse practitioners*. (2nd ed., pp. 265-275). St. Louis, MO: Elsevier.

Barkley, Jr., T., Haskin, R., & Tejedor, M. (2001). Practice issues: Credentialing, prescriptive authority and liability. *Nurse Practitioner Forum, 12*(2), 106-114.

Barkley, Jr., T., & Myers, C. M. (2008). *Practice guidelines for acute care nurse practitioners* (2nd ed.). St. Louis, MO: Elsevier.

Barkley, Jr., T., & Myers, C. M. (2008). Pulmonary function testing. In T. W. Barkley, Jr. & C. M. Myers (Eds.), *Practice guidelines for acute care nurse practitioners* (2nd ed., pp. 259-264). St. Louis, MO: Elsevier.

Barkley, Jr., T., & Rogers, J. E. (2001). Dynamic roles and scope of practice for the acute care nurse practitioner. *Nurse Practitioner Forum, 12*(2), 115-120.

Barkley, Jr., T., Schulman, L. M., & Lopez, J. (2008). HIV/AIDS and opportunistic infections. In T. W. Barkley, Jr. & C. M. Myers (Eds.), *Practice guidelines for acute care nurse practitioners* (2nd ed., pp. 621-631). St. Louis, MO: Elsevier.

Baroni, M. A. (2004). Human growth and development. In V. L. Millonig, M. A. Baroni & B. Bigler (Eds.), *Pediatric nurse practitioner certification review guide* (4th ed.). Potomac, MD: Health Leadership Associates.

Barry, E., Bellgrove, M. A., Cox, M., Hill, M., Johnson, D. A., Kelly S. P., & Robertson, I. H. (2007). Response variability in attention deficit hyperactivity disorder: Evidence for neuropsychological heterogeneity. *Neuropsychologia, 45*(4), 630-638.

Beers, M. H., Jones, T. V., & Porter, R. S. (2006). *The Merck manual of diagnosis and therapy* (18th ed.). Whitehouse Station, NJ: Merck Company.

Behrman, B. E., Jensen, H. B., & Kliegman, R. M. (2011). *Nelson textbook of pediatrics* (19th ed.). Philadelphia, PA: W. B. Saunders.

Berman, S. M., & Workowski, K. A. (2006). Centers for disease control and prevention division of STD prevention. *Sexually transmitted diseases treatment guidelines, 2006.*55(RR11); 1-94. Retrieved from http://www.cdc.gov/mmwr/preview/mmwrhtml/ rr5511a1.htm.

Bickley, L. S., & Szilagyi, P. G. (2008). *Bates' guide to physical examination and history taking,* (10th ed.). Philadelphia, PA: Lippincott.

Birrer, R. B., & O'Connor, F. G. (2004). *Pediatric sports medicine for the primary care physician* (3rd ed.). Boca Raton, FL: CRC Press.

Blair, J., & Selekman, J. (2004). Epilepsy. In P. L. Jackson & J. A. Vessey (Eds.), *Primary care of the child with a chronic condition* (4th ed., pp. 469-497). St. Louis, MO: Mosby.

Blanchard, D. S., & Vermilya, H. L. (2007). Bed sharing. *Holistic Nursing Practice, 21*(1), 1925.

Brashers, V. L. (2006). Clinical application of pathophysiology: An *evidence-based approach* (3rd ed.). St. Louis, MO: Mosby.

Broome, B. S. (2008). Major causes of mortality in the United States. In T. W. Barkley, Jr., & C. M. Myers (Eds.), *Practice guidelines for acute care nurse practitioners* (2nd ed., pp. 931-938). St. Louis, MO: Elsevier.

Broome, B. S., & Barkley Jr., T. W. (2001). Decoding the meaning of research: Applications in acute care. *Nurse Practitioner Forum, 12*(3), 127-137.

Buppert, C. (2008). *Nurse practitioner's business practice and legal guide* (3rd ed.). Sudbury, MA: Jones & Bartlett Publishers.

Buppert. C. (2006). Billing "incident to" when an established patient has a new problem. Retrieved from http://www.buppert.com/ articles/incident-to.php.

Buppert, C. (2006). How to fire a patient. Retrieved from http://www.buppert.com/articles/fire-patient.php.

Buppert, C. (2006). What to do when health plans are vague about policies on NPs. Retrieved from http://www.buppert.com/articles/vague-policy-issues.php.

Buppert, C. (2006). When is a physician liable for nurse practitioner malpractice. Retrieved from http://www.buppert.com/articles/liability.php.

Buppert, C. (2002). NP Services: Reimbursement basics-the Payers. Retrieved from http://medscape.com/ viewarticle 422935 print.

Burke, M. R. (2003). Billing medicare for the services of NP's and PA's. Retrieved from http://www.Physiciansnews.com/business/403burke.html.

Burns, C. E., Brady, M., Blosser, C., & Dunn, A. M. (2004). *Pediatric primary care: A handbook for nurse practitioners* (3rd ed.). Philadelphia, PA: W. B. Saunders.

Burns, C. E. & Dunn, A. M. (2008). *Pediatric primary care* (4th ed.). Philadelphia, PA: Saunders.

Burns, C. E., Dunn, A. M., Brady, M. A., Starr, N. B., & Blosser, C. G. (2008). *Pediatric primary care* (4th ed.).

St. Louis, MO: Saunders.

Burns. C. E., Richardson V., & Brady, M. (2009). *Pediatric primary care case studies.* Jones & Bartlett Publishers, Canada.

Busby, L. C. (2005). Advanced practice trends/issues and health policy. In V. L. Millonig (ed.). *Adult nurse practitioner certification review guide* (4th ed.). Potomac, MD: Health Leadership Associates.

Cady, R. F. (2003). *The advanced practice nurse's legal handbook.* Philadelphia, PA: Lippincott Williams & Wilkins.

Carey, W., Crocker A., Coleman, E. E., & Feldman, H. (2009). *Developmental behavioral pediatrics* (4th ed.). Saunders.

Carol D., & Berkowitz, M. D. (2008). *Berkowitz's pediatrics: A primary care approach* (3rd ed.). Elk Grove Village, IL: American Academy of Pediatrics.

Carroll-Pankhurst, C., & Mortimer, Jr., S. A. (2001). Sudden infant death syndrome, bed sharing, parental weight, and age at death. *Pediatrics, 107*(3), 530-536.

Centers for Disease Control and Prevention (CDC). (2000). Preventing pneumococcal disease among infants and young children: Recommendations of the advisory committee on immunization practices. *Morbidity and Mortality Weekly Report, 49*(RR-9;1), 1-38. Atlanta, GA: Author.

Centers for Disease Control and Prevention (CDC). (2000). Recommendation for blood lead screening of young children enrolled in Medicaid: Targeting a group at high risk. *Morbidity and Mortality Weekly Report, 49*(RR14;1), 1-38. Atlanta, GA: Author.

Centers for Disease Control and Prevention (CDC). (2003). Managing acute gastroenteritis among children: Oral rehydration, maintenance and nutritional therapy (American Academy of Pediatrics Policy). *Morbidity and Mortality Weekly Report, 52*(RR-16), 1-16. Atlanta, GA: Author.

Centers for Disease Control and Prevention (CDC). (2006). *Sexually transmitted diseases treatment guidelines 2006.* Atlanta, GA: Author.

Centers for Disease Control and Prevention (CDC). (2006). Diagnosis and management of tickborne rickettsial diseases: Rocky mountain spotted fever, ehrlichioses, and anaplasmosis: A practical guide for physicians and other health-care and public health professionals in United States. *Morbidity and Mortality Weekly Report, 55*(RR-4); 1-27. Atlanta, GA: Author.

Centers for Disease Control and Prevention (CDC). (2006). Influenza vaccination of health-care personnel: Recommendations of the healthcare infection control practices advisory committee (HICPAC) and the advisory committee on immunization practices (ACIP). *Morbidity and Mortality Weekly Report, 55*(RR-2); 1-16. Atlanta, GA: Author.

Centers for Disease Control and Prevention. (2006). *Contraindications to vaccines chart.* Retrieved from http://www.cdc.gov/nip/recs/contraindications.pdf.

Christman, L. (2004). Leadership roles and management functions in nursing theory and application. *Nursing Administration Quarterly, 28*(3), 225.

Dains, J., Baumann, L. C., & Scheibel P. (2007). *Advanced health assessment and clinical diagnosis in primary care* (3rd ed.). St. Louis, MO: Mosby.

D'Augustine, S., & Flosi, T. (2010). *Tarascon pediatric outpatient pocketbook.* Sudbury, MA: Jones & Bartlett Learning.

Dale, J. C. (2004). Hematological/oncological/immunological disorders. In Millonig, V. L., Baroni, M. A., & Bigler, B. (Eds.), *Pediatric nurse practitioner certification review guide* (4th ed.). Potomac, MD: Health Leadership Associates.

Davis, M., Gruskin, K., & Chang, V. (2004). *Signs and symptoms in pediatrics.* Philadelphia, PA: Mosby.

Davis, R. Q. (2007). The diaper-free baby: The natural toilet training alternative. *Library Journal, 132*(1), 138-139.

Dipiro, J. T., Talbert, R. L., & Yee, G. C. (2008). *Pharmacotherapy: a pathophysiological approach* (7th ed.). New York: McGraw-Hill.

Dixon, S. D., & Stein, M. T. (2006). *Encounters with children: pediatric behavior and development* (4th ed.). St. Louis, MO: Mosby Inc.

Duderstadt, K. (2006). *Pediatric physical examination: An illustrated handbook.* St. Louis, MO: Mosby.

Dusenbery, S. M., & White, A. (2009). *The Washington manual® of pediatrics.* Philadelphia, PA: Lippincott Williams & Wilkins.

Emans S. J., Laufer M. R., & Goldstein D. P. (2004). *Pediatric & adolescent gynecology* (4th ed.). Lippincott Williams & Wilkins.

Escott-Stump, S. (2011). *Nutrition and diagnosis-related care* (7th ed.). Philadelphia, PA: Lippincott Williams & Wilkins.

Ferri, F. F. (2010). *Practical guide to care of the medical patient* (8th ed.). St. Louis, MO: Mosby.

Ferri, F. F. (2009). *Ferri's clinical advisor: Instant diagnosis and treatment* (11th ed.). St. Louis, MO: Mosby.

Fischbach, F., & Dunning M. B. (2008). *A manual of laboratory & diagnostic tests* (8th ed.). Philadelphia, PA: Lippincott Williams & Wilkins.

Flagg, J. S., & Sloand, E. (2010). *Pediatric nurse practitioner certification review guide: Primary care* (5th ed.). Sudbury, MA: Jones & Bartlett Publishers.

Fleisher, R. G., & Ludwig, S (2010). *Textbook of pediatric emergency medicine* (6th ed.). Philadelphia, PA: Lippincott Williams & Wilkins.

Fowler, A. A., & Wenzel, R. P. (2006). Acute bronchitis. *The New England Journal of Medicine, 355*(20), 2125-2130.

Fox, J. A. (2002). *Primary health care of infants, children, and adolescents* (2nd ed.). St. Louis, MO: Mosby.

Frakes, E., & Tracylain, M. A., (2006). *An overview of medicare reimbursement: Regulations for advanced practice nurses.* Retrieved from http://www.redorbit.com/news/health/473424/an_overview_of_medicare_reimbursement_regulations_for_advanced_practice_nurses/index.html?source=r_health.

Frank, G., & Zaoutis, L. (2005). *The Philadelphia guide: Inpatient pediatrics.* Philadelphia, PA: Lippincott Williams & Wilkins.

Friedman, M. M., Bowden, V. R., & Jones, E. G. (2003). *Family nursing: Research, theory and practice* (5th ed.). Upper Saddle River, NJ: Pearson Education.

Gantz, N. R., Sorenson, L., & Howard, R. L. (2003). A Collaborative perspective on nursing leadership in quality improvement: The foundation for outcomes management. *Nursing Administration Quarterly, 27*(4), 324-330.

Garfunkel, L. C., Christy, C., & Kaczorowski, J. (2007). *Mosby's pediatric clinical advisor: Instant diagnosis and treatment* (2nd ed.). St. Louis, MO: Mosby.

Gilbert, D. N. (2010). *The Sanford guide to antimicrobial therapy* (39th ed.). Hyde Park, VT: Antimicrobial Therapy, Inc.

Goroll, A. H., & Mulley, A. G. (2009). *Primary care medicine: Office evaluation and management of the adult patient* (6th ed.). Philadelphia, PA: Lippincott, William & Wilkins.

Graham, M. V., & Uphold, C. R. MV. (2004). *Clinical guidelines in child health* (3rd ed). Gainesville, FL: Barmarrae Books.

Green, M., & Palfrey, J. S. (2008). *Bright futures: Guidelines for health supervision of infants, children, and adolescents* (3rd ed.). Arlington, VA: National Center for Education in Maternal Child Health.

Gunn, V. L., & Nechyba, C. (2002). *Johns Hopkins hospital-children's medical and surgical center. The Harriet Lane handbook, a manual of pediatric house officers* (16th ed). Philadelphia, PA: C. V. Mosby.

Guyton, A. L., & Hall, J. H. (2010). *Textbook of medical physiology* (12th ed.). Philadelphia, PA: Saunders.

Hagan, J. F., Shaw, J. S., & Duncan, P. (2008). *Bright futures: Guidelines for health supervision of infants, children, and adolescents* (3rd ed.). Elk Grove Village, IL: American Academy of Pediatrics.

Hamric, A. B., Spross, J. A., & Hanson, C. (2008*). Advanced practice nursing: An integrative approach* (4th ed.). Philadelphia, PA: Saunders.

Harris, S., & Anderson S. J. (2009). *American academy of pediatrics and American academy of orthopedic surgeons, care of the young athlete* (2nd ed.). AAOS.

Hatcher, R. A., Zieman, M., Cwiak, C., Darney, P. D., Creinen, M. D., & Stosur, H. R. (2010). *A pocket guide to managing contraception 2010-2012.* New York, NY: Ardentmedia, Inc.

Hatcher, R. A., Trussell J., Nelson A. L., Cates W., Stewart F. (2008) *Contraceptive technology (*19th ed.). New York, NY: Contraceptive Technology Communications.

Hay, W., & Levin, M. (2008). *Current diagnosis and treatment pediatrics* (19th ed.). Chicago, IL: McGraw-Hill Medical.

Hay, W. W., Hayward, A. R., Levin, M., Hay, Jr., W. W., & Sondheimer, J. M. (2010). *Current pediatric diagnosis and treatment* (20th ed.). Norwalk, CT: McGraw-Hill/Appleton & Lange.

Hill, N. H., & Sullivan, L. (2004). *Management guidelines for nurse practitioners working with children and adolescents* (2nd ed.). Philadelphia, PA: F. A. Davis.

Heighway, S. (2004). Musculoskeletal disorders. In Millonig, V. L., Baroni, M. A., & Bigler, B. (Eds.), *Pediatric nurse practitioner certification review guide* (4th ed.). Potomac, MD: Health Leadership Associates.

Heighway, S. (2004). Neurological disorders. In Millonig, V. L., Baroni, M. A., & Bigler, B. (Eds.), *Pediatric nurse practitioner certification review guide* (4th ed.). Potomac, MD: Health Leadership Associates.

Hickey, J. V., Ouimette, R. M., & Venegoni, S. L. (2000). *Advanced practice nursing: Changing roles and clinical applications* (2nd ed.) Philadelphia, PA: Lippincott, Williams & Wilkins.

Hudson, C. T., & Dixon, D. (2003). Autism: Challenges in diagnosis and treatment. *Clinician Reviews, 13*, 46-51.

Huether, S. E., & McCance, K. L. (2008). *Advanced practice nursing: Changing roles and clinical applications* (4th ed.). St. Louis, MO: Mosby.

Hughes, S. (2007). HIV and pregnancy: Twenty-five years into the epidemic. *International Anesthesiology, 45*(1), 29-33.

Jackson, Allen P. & Vassey, J. A. (2009). *Primary care of the child with a chronic condition* (5th ed.). Mosby Elsevier.

Jarvis, C. (2008). *Physical examination and health assessment* (5th ed.). St. Louis, MO: Saunders.

Jellinek, M. S. (2002). *Bright futures in practice: Mental health*. Arlington, VA: National Center for Education in Maternal Child Health.

Joint National Committee on Prevention, Detection, Evaluation, and Treatment of High Blood Pressure (JNC). (2004). *7th Report of the JNC*. Washington, DC: National Institutes of Health.

Johnson, K., Hallsey, D., Meredith, R.L., & Warden, E. (2006). A nurse-driven system for improving patient quality outcomes. *Journal of Nursing Care Quality, 21*(2),168-175.

Jones, K. L. (2005). *Smith's recognizable patterns of human malformation* (6th ed.). Philadelphia, PA: W. B. Saunders.

Joseph, Jr., F., & Hagan, M. D. (2007). *Bright futures: Guidelines for health supervision of infants, children, and adolescents* (3rd ed.). Elk Grove Village, IL: American Academy of Pediatrics.

Kanegan, G. V. (2006). Successful management in primary care-depression and anxiety. *Advance for Nurse Practitioners, 14*(10), 79.

King, CK, Glass, R., Bresee, J. S., & Duggan C. (2003). *Managing acute gastroenteritis among children: Oral rehydration, maintenance and nutritional therapy*. MMWR Recomm Rep. 52:1-16.

Kleinpell, R. M., & Hravnak, M. M. (2005). Strategies for success in the acute care nurse practitioner role. *Critical Care Nursing Clinics of North America, 17*(2), 177-81.

Kliegman, R. M., Behman R. E., Henson, H. B., Stanton, B. F. (2011) *Nelson textbook of pediatrics* (19th ed.). Philadelphia, PA: Saunders, Elsevier.

Klish, W. J. (1998). Childhood obesity. *Pediatrics in Review, 19,* 312-315.

Lang, N. M., & Kizer, K. W. (2005). Nursing-sensitive quality performance measures: A key to health care improvement. *AAACN Viewpoint, 27*(2), 1, 8-11.

Lawrence, R. A., & Lawrence, R. M. (2011). *Breastfeeding: A guide for the medical profession* (7th ed.). St. Louis, MO: Mosby-Year Book.

Lithgow, D. I., & Kleinpell, R. M. (1999). Roles, issues, policies, and trends. In A. Gawlinski and D. Hamwi (Eds.), *American association of critical care nurses acute care nurse practitioner clinical curriculum and certification review.* Philadelphia, PA: W. B. Saunders.

Love, S. R. (2008). Anemias. In T. W. Barkley, Jr. and C. M. Myers (Eds.), *Practice guidelines for acute care nurse practitioners* (2nd ed., pp. 541-556). St. Louis, MO: Elsevier.

Love, S. R. (2008). Headaches. In T. W. Barkley, Jr. and C. M. Myers (Eds.), *Practice guidelines for acute care nurse practitioners* (2nd ed., pp. 698-714). St. Louis, MO: Elsevier.

Love, S. R. (2008). Leukemias. In T. W. Barkley, Jr. and C. M. Myers (Eds.), *Practice guidelines for acute care nurse practitioners* (2nd ed., pp. 573-583). St. Louis, MO: Elsevier.

Love, S. R. (2008). Lymphoma. In T. W. Barkley, Jr. and C. M. Myers (Eds.), *Practice guidelines for acute care nurse practitioners* (2nd ed., pp. 584-594). St. Louis, MO: Elsevier.

Love, S. R. (2008). Other common cancers. In T. W. Barkley, Jr. and C. M. Myers (Eds.), *Practice guidelines for acute care nurse practitioners* (2nd ed., pp. 595-620). St. Louis, MO: Elsevier.

Love, S. R. (2008). Sickle cell disease/crisis. In T. W. Barkley, Jr. and C. M. Myers (Eds.), *Practice guidelines for acute care nurse practitioners* (2nd ed., pp. 557-561). St. Louis, MO: Elsevier.

Marcdante, K. (2010). *Nelson essentials of pediatrics.* (6th ed.). Philadelphia, PA: Saunders.

McCance, K. L., Huether, S. E. (2006). *Pathophysiology: The biologic basis for disease in adults and children.* (5th ed.). St. Louis, MO: Mosby Inc.

McInerny, K. T. & Adam, H. M. (2008). *AAP Textbook of pediatric care.* Elk Grove Village, IL: American Academy of Pediatrics.

McInerny, T., Adam H., Campbell D., Kamat D. and Kelleher (2008). AAP *Textbook of pediatric care.* American Academy of Pediatrics.

Melnyk, B. M. (2004). Health maintenance and promotion. In Millonig, V. L., Baroni, M. A., & Bigler, B. (Eds.), *Pediatric nurse practitioner certification review guide* (4th ed.). Potomac, MD: Health Leadership Associates.

Meyer, T. (2008). The chest x-ray. In T.W. Barkley, Jr., & C. M. Myers (Eds.), *Practice guidelines for acute care nurse practitioners.* (2nd ed., pp. 246-252). St. Louis, MO: Elsevier.

Michel, R. S. (1999). Toilet training. *Pediatrics in Review, 20*, 240-245.

Millonig, V. L. (2001). Pediatric *nurse practitioner certification review manual.* Potomac, MD: Health Leadership Associates.

Millonig, V. L. (2005). *Adult nurse practitioner certification review guide.* (4th ed.). Potomac, MD: Health leadership Associates, Inc.

Mirr Jansen, M. P., & Zwygart-Stauffacher, M. (2005). *Advanced practice nursing: Core concepts for professional role development* (3rd ed.). New York, NY: Springer Publishing Company.

Mobley, C., Millonig, V. L., Bigler, B. (2004). *Pediatric nurse practitioner certification review guide* (4th ed.). Sudbury, MA: Jones & Bartlett Publishers.

Moore, K. J. (1998). Billing for NP Services. What you need to know. Retrieved from http://www.aafp.org.fpm/980500fm/billing.html.

Myers, C. M. (2008). Anatomical intestinal disorders. In T. W. Barkley, Jr. & C. M. Myers (Eds.), *Practice guidelines for acute care nurse practitioners* (2nd ed., pp. 392-396). St. Louis, MO: Elsevier.

Myers, C. M. (2008). Biliary dysfunction. In T. W. Barkley, Jr. & C. M. Myers (Eds.), *Practice guidelines for acute care nurse practitioners* (2nd ed., pp. 374-381). St. Louis, MO: Elsevier.

Myers, C. M. (2008). Central nervous system disorders. In T. W. Barkley, Jr. & C. M. Myers (Eds.), *Practice guidelines for acute care nurse practitioners* (2nd ed., pp. 63-71). St. Louis, MO: Elsevier.

Myers, C. M. (2008). Gastrointestinal bleeding. In T. W. Barkley, Jr. & C. M. Myers (Eds.), *Practice guidelines for acute care nurse practitioners* (2nd ed., pp. 397-408). St. Louis, MO: Elsevier.

Myers, C. M. (2008). Inflammatory gastrointestinal disorders. In T. W. Barkley, Jr. & C. M. Myers (Eds.), *Practice guidelines for acute care nurse practitioners* (2nd ed., pp. 382-391). St. Louis, MO: Elsevier.

Myers, C. M. (2008). Liver disease. In T. W. Barkley, Jr. & C. M. Myers (Eds.), *Practice guidelines for acute care nurse practitioners* (2nd ed., pp. 362-373). St. Louis, MO: Elsevier.

Myers, C. M. (2008). Peptic ulcer disease. In T. W. Barkley, Jr. & C. M. Myers (Eds.), *Practice guidelines for acute care nurse practitioners* (2nd ed., pp. 347-361). St. Louis, MO: Elsevier.

Myers, C. M. (2008). Seizure disorders. In T. W. Barkley, Jr. and C. M. Myers (Eds.), *Practice guidelines for acute care nurse practitioners* (2nd ed., pp. 72-81). St. Louis, MO: Elsevier.

National Asthma Education and Prevention Program (2007). *Expert panel report 3: Guidelines for the diagnosis and management of asthma-full report.* Bethesda, MD: National Institute of Health.

National Heart, Lung and Blood Institute (2007). *Expert panel report 3 (EPR3): Guidelines for the diagnosis and management of asthma.* Washington, DC: National Institutes of Health.

National Institutes of Mental Health (2008). *Attention deficit hyperactivity disorder.* Retrieved from http//209.85.173.104/search/q=cache:BNDTk_7ILiUJ:www.nimh.nih.gov/health/publications/adhd/complete publication.shtml+National+Institutes+of+Mental+Health+Attention+deficit+hyperactivity+disorder.&hl=en&ct=clnk&cd=2&gl=us.

National Joint Committee on Learning Disabilities (2006). *Learning disabilities and young children: Identification and intervention.* Retrieved from www.ldonline.org/module=uploads&func=download&fileId=602.

Neinstein, L. S. (2008). *Adolescent health care: A practical guide* (5th ed.). Philadelphia, PA: Lippincott, Williams and Wilkins.

Newby,.J.(2007). Billing services performed by Nurse Practitioners and Physician Assistants. Retrieved from http:www.in-afp.org/files/publicincident_to_Services.

Osborn, L., Dewitt T., First L., & Zenel J. (2004). *Pediatrics.* Philadelphia, PA: Elsevier Mosby.

Parker, S., & Zuckerman, B. (2005). *Behavioral and developmental pediatrics: A handbook for primary care* (2nd ed.). Philadelphia, PA: Lippincott, Williams and Wilkins.

Patrick, K., Spear, B., Holt, K., & Sofka, D. (2002). *Bright futures in practice: Physical activity.* Arlington, VA: National Center for Education in Maternal Child Health.

Paul, D., & Chan, M. D. (2006). *Pediatrics 2007.* Mission Viejo, CA: Current Clinical Strategies.

Pearson, L. (2000). Annual update of how each state stands on legislative issues affecting advanced nursing practice. *Nurse Practitioner, 25*(1).

Pearson, L. (2004) Sixteenth Annual Legislative Update: How each state stands on legislative issues affecting advanced nursing practice. *Nurse Practitioner, 29*(1), 26-51.

Penas, C. D., & Barkley, Jr., T. (2001). Ethical theory and principles of decision making for the acute care nurse practitioner. *Nurse Practitioner Forum, 12*(3), 161-165.

Pickering, L. K., Baker, C. J., Kimberlin, D. W., & Long, S. S. (2009). *Red Book: 2009 report of the committee on infectious diseases.*(28th ed.). Elk Grove Village, IL: American Academy of Pediatrics.

Polin, R. A., & Ditmar, M. F. (2010). *Pediatric secrets* (5th ed.) St. Louis, MO: Mosby.

Polit, D., & Beck, C. T. (2007). *Nursing research: Principles and methods.* (8th ed.). Philadelphia, PA: Lippincott, Williams & Wilkins.

Pollack, J. S., & Daley, A. M. (2003). Improve adolescents' access to emergency contraception. *The Nurse Practitioner, 28*(8), 11.

Prasad, P. (2009). *Pocket pediatrics: The Massachusetts general hospital for children handbook of pediatrics.* Philadelphia, PA: Lippincott, Williams & Wilkins.

Premawardhana, L. D., & Lazarus, J. H. (2006). Management of thyroid disorders. *Postgraduate Medical Journal, 82*(971), 552-558.

Priest, A. (2006). *Bridging the gap between acute care and community care.* New York, NY: Nursing BC.

Public Health Service. (2006). *Healthy people 2010: Understand and improving health* (2nd ed.). Washington, DC: Government Printing Office.

Ramadan, H. H., Lippincott, L., & Brown, K. R. (2006). *Pediatric sinusitis, medical treatment.* Retrieved from http://www.emedicine.com/ent/topic612.htm.

Reilly, J. J., & Wilson, D. (2006). Childhood obesity. *British Medical Journal, 333*(7580), 1207-1210.

Richardson, B. (2005). Practice *guidelines for pediatric nurse practitioners.* St. Louis, MO: Mobsy.

Riley-Bryan, K., & Barkley, Jr., T. (2001). Health policy concerns for the acute care nurse practitioner. *Nurse Practitioner Forum, 12*(2), 98-105.

Roberts, D. (2004). *The legal side of nursing.* Retrieved from www.medsurgnursing. net.

Robertson, J., & Shilkofski, N. (2008). *The Harriet Lane handbook* (18th ed.). St. Louis, MO: Mosby.

Robertson, D. L., & Kish, C. P. (2001). *Core concepts in advanced practice nursing.* St. Louis, MO: Mosby.

Rundio, Jr., A. (2001a). Continuous quality improvement and problem solving techniques for the acute care nurse practitioner. *Nurse Practitioner Forum, 12*(2), 92-97.

Rundio, Jr., A. (2001b). Reimbursement hieroglyphs for the acute care nurse practitioner. *Nurse Practitioner Forum, 12*(3), 138-146.

Sabella, C., & Robert, J., & Cunningham, R. J. (2009). *The Cleveland clinic intensive review of pediatrics* (3rd ed.). Philadelphia, PA: Lippincott, Williams & Wilkins.

Schober, M., & Affara, F. (2006). *Advanced practice nursing.* Malden, MA: Blackwell Publishing.

Schwartz, M. W., Bell, Jr., L. M., & Bingham, P. M. (2008). *5-Minute pediatric consult* (5th ed.). Philadelphia, PA: Lippincott, Williams and Wilkins.

Scruggs, M. D. (2006). *Pediatric treatment guidelines 2007* Mission Viejo, CA: Current Clinical Strategies.

Simms, M. D., & Schum, R. L. (2000). Preschool children who have atypical patterns of development. *Pediatrics in Review, 21*, 1477-158.

Simon, H. (2007). Birth control options for women. Retrieved from http://adam.about.com/reports/Birth-control-options-for-women.htm.

Skinner, H. B. (2006). *Current diagnosis and treatment in orthopedics* (4th ed.). New York, NY: McGraw-Hill.

Society of Pediatric Nurses, National Association of Pediatric Nurse Practitioners, American Nurses Association (2008). *Pediatric Nursing: Scope and Standards of Practice.* Silver Spring, Md: Nursesbooks.org.

Sondheime, J. (2007). *Current essentials of pediatrics.* Chicago, IL: McGraw-Hill Medical.

Springhouse. (2010). *Pediatric facts made incredibly quick!* (2nd ed.). Philadelphia, PA: Lippincott, Williams & Wilkins.

Stein Pollack, A., & Daley, A. M. (2000). Improve adolescents' access to emergency contraception. *Nurse Practitioner, 28*, 11-23.

Story, M., Holt, K., & Sofka, D. (2011). *Bright futures in practice: Nutrition* (3rd ed.). Arlington, VA: National Center for Education in Maternal Child Health.

Swartz, M. H. (2009). *Textbook of physical diagnosis: History and examination* (6th ed.). Philadelphia, PA: Saunders.

Takemoto, C. K., Hodding, J. H., & Kraus, D. M.(2010). *Pediatric dosage handbook: Including neonatal dosing, drug administration and extemporaneous preparations* (17th ed.). Hudson, OH: Lexi-Comp, Inc.

Therapeutic Research Faculty Staff. (2008). *Natural medicines: Comprehensive database* (10th ed.). Stockton, CA: Therapeutic Research Center.

Thompson, I. E., Melia, K. M., & Boyd, K. M. (2006). *Nursing ethics* (5th ed.). New York, NY: Churchill Livingstone.

Tierney, L. M., McPhee, S.,& Papadakis, M. A. (2010). *Current medical diagnosis and treatment* (50th ed.). New York, NY: Lange/McGraw-Hill.

United States Department of Health & Human Services (2006). *Healthy people 2010: Understanding and improving health and objectives for improving health* (2nd ed.). Washington, DC: Author.

United States Department of Health and Human Services (2005). *Healthy people 2010: Midcourse review.* Washington, DC: Author.

United States Department of Health & Human Services(2000). *Healthy people 2010 volume 2: Objectives for improving health* (2nd ed.). Washington, DC: Author

Uphold, C. R., & Graham, M. V. (2006). *Clinical guidelines in family practice* (4th ed.). Gainesville, FL: Barmarrae Books.

Uzark, K. (2004). Cardiovascular disorders. In Millonig, V., Baroni, M. A., & Bigler, B. (Eds.), *Pediatric nurse practitioner certification review guide* (4th ed.). Potomac, MD: Health Leadership Associates.

Virella, G. (2008). *Schwartz's clinical handbook of pediatrics* (4th ed.). Philadelphia, PA: Lippincott Williams & Wilkins.

Vuckovich, P. (2008). Psychosocial problems in acute care. In T. W. Barkley, Jr., & C. M. Myers, (Eds.), *Practice guidelines for acute care nurse practitioners* (2nd ed., pp. 740-759). St. Louis, MO: Elsevier.

Wallach, J. B. (2007). *Interpretation of diagnostic tests* (8th ed.). Philadelphia, PA: Lippincott, William and Wilkins.

Walsh, C. R. (2008). Fractures. In T. W. Barkley, Jr., & C. M. Myers (Eds.), *Practice guidelines for acute care nurse practitioners* (2nd ed., pp. 524-528). St. Louis, MO: Elsevier.

Walsh, C. R. (2008). Soft tissue injury. In T.W. Barkley, Jr., & C. M. Myers (Eds.), *Practice guidelines for acute care nurse practitioners* (2nd ed., pp. 519-523). St. Louis, MO: Elsevier.

Bibliography

Weill, V. (2004). Gastrointestinal disorders. In Millonig, V. L., Baroni, M. A., & Bigler, B. (Eds.), *Pediatric nurse practitioner certification review guide* (4th ed.). Potomac, MD: Health Leadership Associates.

Weston, W., Lane A., & Morelli J. (2007). *Color Textbook of Pediatric Dermatology.* (4th ed.) Philadelphia, PA: Mosby Elsevier.

White, C. (2008). Guidelines for health promotion and screening. In T. W. Barkley, Jr., & C. M. Myers (Eds.), *Practice guidelines for acute care nurse practitioners* (2nd ed., pp. 913-930). Philadelphia, PA: Elsevier.

Williams, K. (2008). Immunization recommendations. In T. W. Barkley, Jr., & C. M. Myers (Eds.), *Practice guidelines for acute care nurse practitioners* (2nd ed., pp. 939-955). St. Louis, MO: Elsevier.

William, M., & Bell, L. M. (2008). *The 5-Minute pediatric consult* (5th ed.). Philadelphia, PA: Lippincott, Williams & Wilkins.

Zitelli, B. J., & Davis, H.W. (2007). *Atlas of pediatric physical diagnosis* (5th ed.). Philadelphia, PA: Elsevier.

Zitelli, B. J., & Davis, H. W. (2007). *Atlas of pediatric physical diagnosis: Text with online access* (5th ed.). St. Louis, MO: Mosby.

NOTES

NOTES

NOTES

NOTES